TH

DID YOU KNOW

- Americans spend more than $150 million a year on sinus medications—many of which are completely ineffective.

- Some common remedies, including overuse of decongestant sprays, can aggravate your condition.

- Approximately half of all asthma sufferers should take measures to avert sinusitis.

- Many physicians incorrectly diagnose and prescribe for sinus conditions.

- Hundreds of thousands of workdays are lost each year to sinusitis.

- Left untreated, sinusitis can result in severe complications including ocular infection and meningitis.

The future is bright for the tens of millions who suffer from chronic sinusitis. Medical, environmental, and even surgical treatments have advanced so rapidly in recent years that even the most severe cases have new grounds for hope. Packed with practical information, including the most effective home remedies, this up-to-the-minute guide gives you everything *you* need to know.

RELIEF FROM CHRONIC SINUSITIS

THE DELL MEDICAL LIBRARY

THE DELL MEDICAL LIBRARY

Relief from

CHRONIC
SINUSITIS

Marilynn Larkin

Foreword by Howard M. Druce, M.D.

A LYNN SONBERG BOOK

Published by
Dell Publishing
a division of
Bantam Doubleday Dell Publishing Group, Inc.
1540 Broadway
New York, New York 10036

Research about sinusitis is ongoing and subject to interpretation. Although every effort has been made to include the most up-to-date and accurate information about sinusitis in this book, there can be no guarantee that what we know about this complex subject won't change with time. The reader should bear in mind that this book should not be used for self-diagnosis or self-treatment, and appropriate medical professionals should be consulted regarding all health concerns.

ISBN: 0-440-21361-4

Published by arrangement with Lynn Sonberg Book Services, 260 West 72 Street, 6-C, New York, NY 10023

Printed in the United States of America

Published simultaneously in Canada

October 1993

10 9 8 7 6 5 4 3 2 1

OPM

FOREWORD

Sinusitis is among the most prevalent of the chronic diseases. Its symptoms are often debilitating and can interfere with the sinusitis sufferer's ability to work, socialize, and participate in other normal acitvities of daily living. Chronic postnasal drip, nasal secretions, malodorous breath, headache, facial pain, and diminished sense of smell are symptoms that may significantly curtail a person's ability to function and enjoy life. People with asthma are particularly vulnerable to the effects of sinusitis, because recent studies reveal sinusitis may actually trigger asthma attacks.

Increased awareness of the prevalence and potential severity of sinusitis has led to new research on the pathophysiology, diagnosis, and treatment of this disorder. Preliminary data challenge some of the traditional assumptions about the management of this common condition and point to the need for national guidelines. When sinusitis is incorrectly managed, sinus disease is likely to persist, often leading to symptoms that never seem to go away and acute sinus attacks that recur again and again over a period of months or years.

In *Relief from Chronic Sinusitis,* the author presents the latest thinking about how sinusitis develops and how it can be effectively treated. She also explains why sinusitis is often a diagnostic challenge to the physician and reviews the new tools available to help confirm a diagnosis.

The basic message in this book is a positive one: Sinusitis is a controllable disease when treated correctly. Proper medical treatment, often coupled with supportive nonpharmacological strategies such as steam inhalation or saline nasal sprays, can keep sinusitis symptoms from seriously disturbing your quality of life.

Although we still have much to learn about why and how sinuses become inflamed or infected, and the relationship between sinus symptoms and other disorders such as allergies and asthma, *Relief from Chronic Sinusitis* provides a very useful compendium of our current knowledge and can serve as a practical guide to readers who want to help themselves by taking control of sinusitis —by becoming informed, seeking proper treatment, and incorporating some simple supportive therapies into their daily routines.

HOWARD M. DRUCE, M.D.
Clinical Associate Professor of Medicine
Division of Allergy and Immunology
University of Medicine and Dentistry of New Jersey

CONTENTS

ACKNOWLEDGMENTS

The author gratefully acknowledges the generous cooperation and support of the following people: Howard M. Druce, M.D., clinical associate professor of medicine, division of allergy and immunology, University of Medicine and Dentistry of New Jersey, for providing much of the clinical information about sinusitis for this book; David Kennedy, M.D., professor and chairman of the department of otorhinolaryngology—head and neck surgery, University of Pennsylvania, for sharing his expertise on endoscopic surgery for Chapter 6; Harold Nelson, M.D., senior staff physician, National Jewish Center for Immunology and Respiratory Medicine, for providing an overview of sinusitis; and Joseph Abularrage, M.D., chief of pediatrics, Booth Memorial Hospital, and Richard Saphir, M.D., clinical professor of pediatrics, Mount Sinai School of Medicine, for addressing the issue of sinusitis in children.

She also thanks Noah Chivian, D.D.S., spokesperson for the American Association of Endodontists, for providing information on dental disorders and sinusitis; and herbalist Jason Elias, for providing information on herbs and acupressure for Chapter 5.

INTRODUCTION

Sinusitis is one of the most common ailments in the United States today. Consider these facts:

- More than 33 million Americans suffer from chronic sinusitis.

- Sinusitis accounts for approximately 16 million doctor visits annually.

- Americans spend more than $150 million annually for medications prescribed or recommended for the treatment of sinusitis.

- More than 18 percent of adults aged 45 to 64 have sinusitis, or 187 per 1,000 persons.

- Close to 17 percent of adults over age 65 have sinusitis, or 169 per 1,000 persons.

- As many as 10 percent of upper respiratory infections in early childhood are complicated by sinusitis.

- Approximately half of all patients with mild or severe asthma have chronic sinusitis.

- Sinusitis sufferers annually lose hundreds of thousands of days from school and work.

Surprisingly, despite its enormous impact, sinusitis remains largely misunderstood, misdiagnosed, and mismanaged. Even the exact functions of the sinuses themselves —and how sinusitis hampers these functions—aren't completely clear.

Diagnosis is difficult because sinusitis frequently occurs in association with other upper respiratory disorders, such as viral infections or allergies. Symptoms tend to overlap, making it hard to determine which condition is causing problems. What's more, until recently, few diagnostic tools were available to help discover where and why infections occurred.

Additional confusion results from inappropriate treatment of sinusitis. Many people attempt to treat symptoms themselves with over-the-counter products—yet some of these medications do more harm than good. They also won't help cure an active sinus infection, which can occur at any time if you have chronically blocked sinuses. Some physicians are not well versed in the treatment of sinusitis and may prescribe the wrong medicines to treat infection or relieve symptoms, or the appropriate medicines for too short a period of time. As a result, sinusitis becomes prolonged and recurring.

WHY SINUSITIS IS A PROBLEM

Sinusitis is a problem because it undermines your health and can lead to potentially serious complications. When your sinuses are inflamed, you may experience one or more of a wide range of irritating and often painful symptoms: congestion, postnasal drip, cough, yellow or green nasal secretions, bad breath, diminished sense of smell, and varying degrees of headache and facial pain; when active infection sets in on top of chronic inflammation, you may have these symptoms plus sore throat, earache, tooth pain, or fever. These symptoms can cause you to miss work or keep your children home from school.

Even when you feel capable of functioning, you're likely to be continuously aware of annoying symptoms. This constant, low-level irritation can disturb your concentration and make you feel impatient, short-tempered, and generally "stressed out."

If left untreated or treated incorrectly, sinusitis may persist for weeks or months at a time, and sinus infections may recur again and again. Worse, over the long term, sinusitis can cause severe complications such as meningitis or infection of the eye or brain. Recent studies also suggest that sinusitis can trigger severe bronchial asthma attacks.

THE GOOD NEWS ABOUT SINUSITIS

Recent advances in the techniques used to diagnose sinusitis, coupled with improved medications to treat the disorder, have led to much good news about sinusitis. Today, physicians are better able to view the area where the sinuses drain into the nose and throat—known as the *ostiomeatal complex*—the most common site of sinus blockage. Researchers are also gaining a better understanding of how and why these blockages occur. Advances have also been made in sinus surgery, which may be recommended under certain circumstances.

Many of the annoying and debilitating symptoms of sinusitis can now be relieved or eliminated altogether with proper medication. Environmental control—vigorous cleaning and removal of allergens in your home—can reduce sinusitis symptoms associated with allergy. Even home remedies such as steam inhalation and nontraditional herbal remedies are gaining respect as supportive treatments, to be used in conjunction with prescribed medication to help relieve symptoms.

Simply put, the good news about sinusitis is this: You don't have to suffer needlessly from persistent sinus infections. By reading this book and enlisting the help of an experienced physician, you can join the millions of people who have said, "I never realized how bad I was feeling *before* I went to the doctor—until *after* my sinusitis was successfully treated!"

WHY YOU NEED THIS BOOK

Relief from Chronic Sinusitis can help you in three important ways. First, it guides you through the often complicated process of diagnosing sinusitis and determining which conditions—for example, allergy, viral or bacterial infection, stress, nasal polyps, deviated septum, dental disorders, cigarette smoke, and more—predispose you to sinus attacks.

This book also contains explanations of the physiology of the sinuses and of the interactions among the sinuses, nose, teeth, and other structures in the head. Understanding how problems in these areas can affect the sinuses—and vice versa—helps clarify why certain symptoms occur.

Finally, *Relief from Chronic Sinusitis* presents the latest thinking about the treatment of sinusitis. You'll learn which medications work and which don't, when to consider surgery, and what you can do on your own to reduce sinusitis symptoms. This book also provides sources of additional help and information.

In Chapter 1, you'll learn about normal sinuses and what happens when they become inflamed and infected. You'll also learn about complications that can develop from sinusitis.

Chapter 2 explores the conditions that cause increased susceptibility to sinusitis, such as colds, allergies, stress, overuse of decongestant sprays, and structural problems in the nose.

Chapter 3 addresses the issue of diagnosis, including how doctors differentiate between sinusitis and allergic disorders. This chapter also discusses the use of computed tomography (CT) scans and other techniques for visualizing the sinuses, and the role of the *endoscope*—a tubelike instrument with a lens, light source, and sometimes tiny surgical instruments attached to it—in viewing the ostiomeatal complex. You'll also learn how to choose a doctor who is knowledgeable about the latest diagnostic techniques.

Chapter 5 covers medical treatment of sinusitis and of disorders that lead to sinusitis, such as allergies and structural problems in the nose. The importance of selecting a pharmacist who can help explain and coordinate your medications is also discussed.

Chapter 5 covers nonmedical techniques for relieving symptoms, including environmental control, the role of healthful eating and regular exercise, home remedies, herbal treatments, acupressure, and relaxation techniques. These strategies can be helpful when used in addition to—not instead of—medical therapy.

Should you undergo sinus surgery? This is the topic of Chapter 6, which explains when surgery may be appropriate and what to expect.

Chapter 7 discusses how sinusitis affects children. It includes guidelines for parents, which can make diagnosing and treating a child's sinusitis easier and more effective.

Finally, Chapter 8 offers hints and tips for living with sinusitis. It is followed by a section on organizations that can serve as resources and sources of help after you've finished reading this book.

Remember, you don't have to suffer endlessly from the stressful symptoms of sinusitis. Recent research on this long-neglected disorder has led to breakthroughs in its diagnosis and treatment. By reading this book, communicating with a knowledgeable physician, following the prescribed treatment plan, and when needed, making some changes in your life-style, you can turn the tables on sinusitis and reduce or eliminate its symptoms entirely.

Now turn the page and take your first steps toward breaking the cycle of chronic sinusitis.

ONE

WHAT IS SINUSITIS?

Feel congested when you wake up in the morning? Do you have a postnasal drip? Headache? A feeling of "fullness" in your face, especially in the cheek area and under your eyes? If the answer is yes, you may be suffering from sinusitis.

Simply put, *sinusitis* is "an inflammation of a sinus." But as many sinusitis sufferers know, this simple definition gives little indication of the misery and pain caused by the disease, especially when chronically inflamed sinuses become actively infected. In order to understand how and why sinusitis and its symptoms develop, it helps to know something about how healthy sinuses function and how the sinuses are affected by what goes on in the nose and teeth. It's also important to know about the possible complications of sinusitis.

WHAT ARE THE SINUSES?

A sinus is a hollow air space, of which there are many in the body. But when we talk about having a "sinus attack," we're referring to problems in one or more of the four pairs of air spaces known as the *paranasal sinuses* (*para* = "near"; *nasal* = "nose"). These sinuses are located in the bones of the face and head that surround and connect with the nasal cavity (*cavity* is another anatomic word for a hollow air space—in this case, the space that makes up the inner part of the nose).

The sinuses are named for the bone or bones in which they lie. The *frontal sinuses* are located in the brow area, directly over the eyes. The *maxillary sinuses* are inside each cheekbone. The *ethmoid* sinuses are located right behind the bridge of the nose, and the *sphenoid* sinuses are just behind the ethmoids, in the upper part of the nose.

The sinuses have openings on the side of the nose, known as *ostia,* through which mucus drains.

The sinuses are lined with the same kinds of cells and glands as the ones that line the nose. These cells are called *columnar epithelial cells*—epithelial cells that are shaped like columns. When sinusitis is left untreated or treated incorrectly, these cells may become irreversibly damaged.

Each epithelial cell has approximately 25 hairlike projections called *cilia* extending from the top. In healthy sinuses, these cilia are in a constant state of sweeping motion. When the sinuses become infected and inflamed, the sweeping movement of the cilia decreases or may even stop altogether.

The cilia are covered by a blanket of mucus produced by mucous glands in the lining of the sinuses. When the sinuses are infected, the normally clear mucus becomes filled with pus, creating what is known as *mucopus.*

The Sinuses

Ethmoid sinus

Maxillary sinus

Frontal sinus

Sphenoid sinus

Maxillary sinus

Front View

Ethmoid sinus

Frontal sinus

Maxillary sinus

Side View

WHAT IS THE JOB OF THE SINUSES?

Amazingly, despite many years of research, the functions of the paranasal sinuses are not completely understood. Most scientists agree that the sinuses help lighten the weight of the skull and give resonance to the voice (think of how "heavy" your head feels when your sinuses are clogged—and how your voice may sound "thinner" than usual). The sinuses may also play a role in our sense of smell and in warming and humidifying the air we breathe, which are functions that are also performed by the nose.

But the most important job of the sinuses is believed to be their ability to produce a protective mucous blanket. This mucous blanket traps disease-causing microorganisms and foreign particles that escape filtration by the nose.

HOW DO HEALTHY SINUSES WORK?

In healthy sinuses, the openings (ostia) that lead into the nose are unobstructed. This means that the mucus produced in the sinuses drains freely into the nose, carrying with it viruses, bacteria, and other infectious microorganisms, as well as irritants and debris. The mucus is then swept to the back of the nose and swallowed.

The maxillary sinuses, frontal sinuses, and part of the ethmoid sinuses drain into the nose through an opening in the part of the inner nose known as the *middle meatus* (*meatus* is yet another anatomic word for a space or opening, just like *sinus* and *ostium*). The middle meatus is located under a fingerlike extension in the inner nose called the *middle turbinate.* The remaining part of the ethmoid sinuses and the sphenoid sinuses drain into openings in or near the *superior meatus,* which is located under the superior turbinate.

These structures and openings become important when you have sinusitis. Sometimes the middle turbinate or superior turbinate becomes so swollen that the meatus is hidden and blocked. As we'll soon see, this is one of the conditions that can lead to sinusitis.

HOW DOES THE NOSE AFFECT THE SINUSES?

Because the nose and the sinuses are so intimately related —anatomically speaking, that is—it's easy to see how an infection or obstruction in the nose can lay the groundwork for clogged sinuses. And in fact, nose problems are among the most common causes of sinusitis. (These causes will be explored in detail in Chapter 2.)

Anything that causes the nose to become stuffed up, such as a cold, allergy, or bacterial infection, is likely to affect the sinuses. When the nose is stuffy, it tends to swell inside, which can result in blocking of the sinus ostia. This sets the stage for infection in the sinuses.

Ironically, attempting to clear up a stuffed nose with a decongestant spray can also lead to sinusitis. Overuse of these sprays actually causes the sinusitis symptoms to recur. This is known as "rhinitis medicamentosa." (See Chapter 2.)

The nose is also the entry point for viruses, bacteria, and other infectious or irritating material. If the nose doesn't filter out these substances, they may find their way up into the sinuses. Normally, these substances are removed in the mucous blanket. But under certain circumstances, they remain in the sinuses and lead to sinus attacks.

Structural problems in the nose such as a deviated septum or bone spurs can interfere with sinus drainage and lay the groundwork for sinusitis. Nasal polyps—balloon-like swellings in the lining of the nose—can also predispose you to sinusitis.

In effect, whenever the normal functioning of the nose is disrupted, sinusitis may develop.

HOW DO THE TEETH AFFECT THE SINUSES?

Up to 25 percent of sinusitis cases that involve the maxillary sinuses may be due to dental infection, according to recent studies. The roots of the canine teeth and the maxillary molar teeth are in close contact with the floor of the sinuses. An inflammation or infection of any of these roots may lead to sinusitis, and symptoms won't clear up until the dental problem is treated.

As we'll see in Chapter 3, if the cause of your sinusitis isn't clear-cut, your dentist may need to examine you to determine whether a tooth problem is the cause of your symptoms.

HOW DOES SINUSITIS DEVELOP?

Here's a look, in simplified form, at how most cases of sinusitis develop:

1. *An irritating or infectious substance enters the nose.* It may be an allergen, a virus, some form of bacteria, a chemical, or some other foreign particle. In response to the infection or irritation, the linings of the nose and sinuses swell up and mucus production increases.

2. *The sinus openings (ostia) become blocked.* The swollen lining of the inner nose blocks the openings through which mucus produced in the sinuses normally drains. The turbinates may also swell up, hiding the sinus openings. The mucus has nowhere to go and begins filling up the sinuses.

3. *Mucus accumulates in the sinuses.* The trapped mucus sits in the sinuses, creating a dark, wet environment with very little oxygen passing through—perfect for the growth of bacteria.

4. *The sweeping motion of the cilia decreases.* The stagnant mucus slows down the sweeping movement of the cilia at the time they are needed most. For mucus to be swept out of the sinuses, the cilia need to beat freely to push the mucus along to the sinus openings. But the accumulation of mucus prevents cilia from performing their normally brisk sweeping action. In some cases, the epithelial cells themselves become damaged by infection. As a result, the cilia may also be damaged.

5. *Mucus becomes infected and forms mucopus.* Mucopus
   —thick green or yellow secretions from the sinuses—
   is one of the common symptoms of sinusitis.

6. *Mucopus further slows down the cilia and causes more
   blockage of the sinus openings.* Thus, a vicious cycle is
   created.

Fortunately, with proper medical treatment, this cycle
can be broken. Once the infected sinuses are cleared and
the ostia are unblocked, in most cases the cilia start beat-
ing regularly again, sweeping mucus out of the sinuses.

The process described above is the way sinusitis occurs
when it is caused by a local condition—that is, some
problem in the nose, teeth, or sinuses themselves. Very
rarely, sinusitis is caused by a systemic condition, such as
a compromised immune system. How these conditions
affect the sinuses is discussed in Chapter 2, along with the
other causes of sinusitis.

ACUTE OR CHRONIC SINUSITIS?

Physicians have different definitions for *acute* and *chronic*
sinusitis. For the purposes of this book, *chronic sinusitis*
refers either to a situation wherein the sinuses remain
inflamed or infected for a long period of time or to a
situation in which you have a series of acute sinus attacks
over a long period of time—that is, your sinuses are inflamed for a week or so; they clear up with or without
medication; a short time later they become inflamed
again; and the pattern repeats itself over and over.

Chronic sinusitis can also refer to cases where your

sinuses become actively infected, you take medicine over the prescribed period of time, and your sinus infection clears up—only to recur again several weeks or months later.

It's important to realize that in chronic sinusitis your sinuses may either be inflamed or infected or both. All three conditions may cause symptoms, but usually symptoms of inflammation are less severe than symptoms of infection. With inflamed sinuses, you may experience a continuous, dull ache in the sinus areas and perhaps headache, cough, postnasal drip, watery sinus secretions, bad breath, and congestion over long periods of time. You may even adapt to the symptoms and figure this is how you are—which is rarely true, since treatments described in Chapters 4 and 5 may well relieve these symptoms.

When your sinuses are actively infected, you may have the symptoms described above plus severe pain in the sinus areas, sharp headache, yellow or green sinus secretions, fever, chills, sore throat, earache, toothache, weakness, and other signs of infection as well as a stuffed nose and congestion. In these cases, you will need to take one or more of the prescription medicines described in Chapter 4 to treat the infection, plus you may take medicine and follow nonmedical treatment strategies for symptom relief.

SYMPTOMS OF SINUSITIS

To summarize, symptoms of chronic sinusitis may include:

_____ Stuffy nose

_____ Diminished sense of smell

_____ Postnasal drip

_____ Bad breath

_____ Cough

_____ Facia! pain

_____ Headache

_____ Yellow or green nasal secretions (usually during active infection)

_____ Toothache

_____ Earache (especially in children)

_____ Fever (usually during active infection)

_____ Sore throat

_____ Fatigue

As you can see, these symptoms are not peculiar to sinusitis; they also commonly occur during a cold, flu, allergy attack, or some other type of inflammation or infection. This often makes it difficult for physicians to accurately diagnose sinusitis and to pinpoint the affected sinuses.

Sometimes the location of an area of pain and tenderness provides a hint as to which sinuses are inflamed. For example, pain and tenderness in the cheek and upper teeth may signal an infection in the maxillary sinus; pain in the forehead, above the eyebrow, can indicate infection of the frontal sinuses; an infected sphenoid sinus may produce pain behind the eyeball; and pain around the eye socket can be a sign of infection of the ethmoid sinus.

But in most instances, sinusitis presents a real diagnostic challenge to physicians—not only because the symptoms are so common and have such varied causes but also because many people suffer from more than one condition simultaneously; for example, they have both sinusitis and an allergy. What physicians do to search beyond the symptoms to make a *differential diagnosis*—distinguishing sinusitis from other causes of symptoms—is explored in Chapter 3.

COMPLICATIONS OF SINUSITIS

Fortunately, when a sinus infection is accurately diagnosed and properly treated, the condition clears up in a vast majority of cases. However, untreated or inappropriately treated sinusitis can cause severe complications. A pus-filled sinus can act as a breeding ground for infection that may extend to nearby structures, including the eye and the brain. Meningitis, brain abscess, infection of the tissue around the eye, and infections of the bones around the sinuses are all potential complications of sinusitis.

Much recent scientific work has also revealed a close connection between sinusitis and bronchial asthma. Sinusitis is a proven trigger of severe asthma attacks, whether sinuses are infected or merely inflamed. If you have sinusitis and asthma, you should have your sinusitis treated promptly and completely. On a positive note, studies have shown that when you have both conditions and sinusitis is correctly treated, asthma is easier to control.

IMPORTANT POINTS ABOUT
SINUSES AND SINUSITIS

- There are four sets of paranasal sinuses: the frontal sinuses, the maxillary sinuses, the ethmoids, and the sphenoids. Any or all of them can become inflamed or infected.

- Healthy sinuses produce a protective blanket of mucus that traps viruses, bacteria, and other potentially harmful substances.

- Hairlike projections called cilia sweep the mucus out through the sinus ostia and into the nose and throat.

- When the nose becomes stuffy and congested, the sinus ostia may become blocked. This sets the stage for sinusitis.

- Problems with the teeth, such as an infected root, can also affect the sinuses.

- In sinusitis, the sinuses become clogged with mucus. The cilia can't do their job of moving the mucus to the ostia. The ostia themselves become blocked, trapping mucus in the sinuses. The sinuses become inflamed or infected, and mucopus forms.

- Sinusitis can cause debilitating symptoms whether sinuses are actively infected or chronically inflamed.

When infection sets in, it must be treated promptly with appropriate medicine.

• Without proper medical treatment, serious complications may occur. With proper treatment, sinusitis can be cured and often prevented from recurring.

Are you at risk for developing chronic sinusitis? In the next chapter, we'll explore the many conditions that can set the stage for sinus problems.

CAUSES OF SINUSITIS

In this chapter, we'll take a closer look at the many medical and environmental conditions that can predispose you to chronic sinusitis.

UPPER RESPIRATORY TRACT INFECTION

Upper respiratory tract infections frequently lower your body's resistance to the viruses, bacteria, and fungi that may cause sinusitis. Healthy people can successfully fend off these disease-causing microorganisms. But when your body is busy fighting a disease that affects your nose and throat, your defense system can be severely taxed. As a result, viruses, bacteria, or fungi have an opportunity to gain a foothold in your clogged sinuses.

Viral Infection

Any virus that enters the body through the nasal passages can set off a chain reaction leading to a sinus attack. Examples include viruses that cause the common cold, flu, and measles—all of which produce congestion and stuffiness in the nose. Once the lining of the nose swells up, the sinus passages become blocked, and mucus accumulates in the sinuses. A secondary bacterial infection may develop in the clogged sinuses, resulting in infectious sinusitis (in this case, sinusitis is called a *secondary infection* because it develops on top of the primary respiratory infection). Or mucus can sit around in the sinuses and become stagnant, which also causes sinusitis symptoms.

Amazingly, any one of more than 200 different types of viruses can cause the common cold and, by extension, trigger sinusitis. For example, a whole family of viruses called *rhinoviruses* is believed to cause a majority of the common cold symptoms that appear in September and October, whereas another family of viruses known as *coronaviruses* causes many of the colds adults suffer in midwinter, according to the National Institute of Allergy and Infectious Diseases. Any one of these viruses may indirectly lead to sinusitis.

How do you know when symptoms such as congestion, stuffiness, sore throat, and nasal discharge are no longer signs of a cold but are in fact signs of sinusitis? Although it's not always easy to tell when a cold has crossed the line into sinusitis, clues include symptoms that recur over and over (that is, you think you're over your "cold"—only to have it come back a day or two later) or symptoms that seem to never quite go away. A rule of thumb is that cold symptoms lasting more than a few weeks may in fact be signs of sinusitis. How physicians distinguish between the two conditions will be covered in detail in the next chapter.

Bacterial Infection

Bacterial infections can also lead to sinusitis. Like viruses, bacteria cause upper respiratory infections that affect the nose and throat and may eventually settle in the sinuses. Common culprits include *Streptococcus* and *Haemophilus influenzae* bacteria.

Normal sinuses contain no bacteria. Only when the sinuses become clogged with mucus do they become a potential breeding ground for bacteria. Most healthy people tolerate a wide variety of bacteria in the upper respiratory tract with no apparent ill effects until the body's defenses are weakened by disease, or drainage from the sinuses is impeded by a cold or other viral infection. Then bacteria that have been lurking harmlessly in the nose and other areas near the sinuses move in and trigger an infection.

Fungal Infection

Fungi occasionally cause infections in the upper respiratory tract of healthy people. But they are more likely to cause sinusitis in someone whose defenses are compromised by a severe viral infection or diseases such as leukemia, uncontrolled diabetes, or acquired immunodeficiency syndrome (AIDS).

ALLERGIC RHINITIS

Sinusitis is a frequent complication of allergic rhinitis, and the two conditions often exist simultaneously. How a physician meets the diagnostic challenge of distinguishing between the two is discussed in Chapter 3.

Hay fever, rose fever, grass fever, and *"summer colds"* are various names for seasonal allergic rhinitis. If you are among the estimated 22 million Americans who suffer from seasonal allergic rhinitis, you are at risk for developing a chronic sinus infection.

Other forms of allergic rhinitis can lead to sinusitis. One is *mold allergy.* Molds are fungi: Outdoors, they grow on dead leaves, grass, straw, and grains; indoors, they grow on houseplants and soil, on food, in damp places such as basements, and on damp clothing where they cause mildew. The outdoor mold season can extend almost year-round, except when there is snow on the ground. Molds can be found indoors year-round, especially in house dust. (Note: Although molds are fungi, they do not cause fungal infections in the sinuses; rather, by triggering an allergic reaction in a susceptible individual, they cause nasal congestion and stuffiness, which in turn can lead to sinus symptoms resulting from inflammation or bacterial infection.)

House dust mites—tiny insects found in house dust along with molds and disintegrating cellulose from furniture stuffing—are another frequent cause of allergic rhinitis in susceptible individuals.

Cockroach allergy is a recently discovered condition that can cause allergic rhinitis. Inhaling the insects' body scales and fecal material can provoke respiratory allergy symptoms.

Animal dander—bits of shedding skin from your pet—can also be responsible for allergic rhinitis.

Environmental irritants may also trigger an allergic reaction, according to the American Academy of Otolaryngology—Head and Neck Surgery. A primary irritant is ozone, the colorless, pungent gas in smog. It is formed at ground level when motor vehicle exhaust and industrial emissions react with sunlight (this pollutant is different from ozone in the upper atmosphere, which is formed naturally and shields the earth from harmful ultraviolet radiation from the sun). High levels of ozone can double an individual's sensitivity to an allergen, the academy reports. Up to 130 million people, or about half of the U.S. population, live in areas where ozone concentrations exceed the maximum safe standard of 0.12 parts per million.

Ozone levels peak in late afternoon, at the height of the time that sunlight and automobile and industrial fumes combine in the air. For people who are allergic, this problem can be especially difficult in the summer, which is the peak season for many airborne allergens.

Sick building syndrome is a commonly used term to describe clusters of symptoms—including allergic reactions—that occur when you work in an insulated building (where windows are sealed shut) or live in a tightly closed, "energy-efficient" home that offers little ventilation. Particles—dust, microorganisms, and chemical vapors from carpeting and furniture, to name a few—overwhelm the respiratory system, making it impossible for the body to filter out all the irritants, thereby contributing to sinusitis.

How Does an Allergy Cause Sinusitis?

An allergic reaction can cause sinusitis because the nasal symptoms associated with the reaction—swelling of the membranes lining the nose, overproduction of mucus— may cause the sinuses to become blocked. As a result, mucus builds up in the sinus cavities. As we saw in Chapter 1, this dark, moist, clogged area is an environment in which inflammation or infection is likely to develop.

Because sinusitis frequently occurs as a consequence of the symptoms of allergy (and may at times be confused with an allergic reaction), it helps to understand the differences between the two.

Sinusitis, as we've seen, is an inflammation or infection of the sinuses that can be triggered by the many factors described in this chapter. An allergic reaction, on the other hand, is a specific immune system response by the body to plant or animal substances that are foreign to humans. These substances are called *allergens*.

Allergens that cause upper respiratory reactions enter the body through the membranes of the eyes, nose, or throat (in most cases, we simply breathe them in). An immune reaction occurs in the body to counteract the invasion of these foreign substances. Normally, this is a helpful response that protects the body by helping to "wash away"—with tears or nose blowing—the irritating substance.

But in some people, the immune reaction becomes exaggerated, and the membranes become inflamed. This happens when the invading allergens stimulate the body to form substances called *sensitizing antibodies*. The allergens and sensitizing antibodies combine, causing the cells that line the nose, eyes, and air passages to release a potent chemical called *histamine*. Histamine triggers swelling of the nasal membranes, which in turn can lead to overproduction of mucus and poor ciliary clearance of mucus from the nose. As we've seen, this sets the stage for clogging of the sinus ostia—and sinusitis.

FOOD ALLERGIES

The link between food allergies and sinusitis is controversial. Some physicians question whether food allergies exist at all; they believe a true allergic reaction, as described above, rarely occurs to substances in food. Instead, they claim that some foods trigger "adverse reactions" that can be caused by either allergic or nonallergic mechanisms. These reactions may include a range of symptoms such as headache, congestion, shortness of breath, sneezing, rashes, cramps, and feelings of anxiety. Other physicians believe that food allergies cause these symptoms and that certain foods can play a role in sinusitis, just as other allergens do.

For the purposes of this book, it doesn't matter whether a person has a true allergic reaction to a specific food or has an adverse reaction to it. With respect to sinusitis, the result is the same: Any food that causes the person who eats it to have a stuffy nose has the potential to cause sinusitis. According to the Asthma and Allergy Foundation of America, up to 25 percent of people who experience a reaction to food also experience respiratory symptoms.

The parts of foods that provoke reactions are usually

proteins that can cause reactions even after being cooked or digested. According to the American Academy of Allergy and Immunology, recent studies indicate that the proteins in cow's milk, eggs, peanuts, wheat, and soy are the most common food substances that trigger allergic or adverse reactions. Also, alcohol can cause nasal membranes to swell and block the sinus ostia.

NONALLERGIC RHINITIS

Numerous conditions that have nothing to do with allergies can trigger nasal symptoms that are similar to those caused by allergic reactions—sneezing, runny nose, sore throat, postnasal drip. Of course, these conditions set the stage for sinusitis as well.

From the point of view of developing sinusitis, it makes no difference whether the condition affecting the nose and sinuses is infectious, allergic, or nonallergic; the result—stuffy nose and clogged sinus ostia—is the same. Identifying the disorder becomes important in the diagnosis stage, however (see the next chapter), because treatment to alleviate symptoms varies, depending on the cause. As you're probably beginning to realize, diagnosing the cause of sinusitis can be very complicated, given all the possible conditions that can lead to sinus inflammation or infection.

Rhinitis Medicamentosa

Paradoxically, a frequent cause of nonallergic rhinitis—and subsequently sinusitis—is overuse of topical decongestants, more commonly known as nasal sprays or nose drops. This happens when you use over-the-counter nasal sprays or nose drops for more than the indicated three-day maximum and end up with *rebound congestion*—that is, you end up more congested than you were with the cold you were trying to treat.

Here's a simplified look at how rebound congestion develops: After a few days of use, a nasal spray starts relieving congestion for shorter and shorter periods of time. In the first few days, it may provide relief for as long as 12 hours. By day four, you may experience relief from congestion for an hour or less at the same dosage. This means you've developed a tolerance for the drug.

The treatment for this situation is to stop using the nasal spray (see Chapter 4). When you do this, your sinus symptoms may recur with a fury. This is called rebound congestion. This rebound effect may lead to sinusitis because it can create severe nasal congestion.

Vasomotor Rhinitis

Also known as *irritant rhinitis,* vasomotor rhinitis is a condition of unknown origin that seems to be triggered by environmental factors such as smoke, fumes, offensive odors, and weather and air pressure changes. This condition is different from allergic rhinitis, which is caused by an allergy to some allergen in the environment. Although symptoms are similar—congestion, runny nose, headache —no *specific* allergen or cause for the reaction can be found. Vasomotor rhinitis usually afflicts adults year-round.

Nonallergic, Eosinophilic Rhinitis

Like vasomotor rhinitis, this condition may be caused by changes in weather or air pressure. It's named for the white blood cell that distinguishes it from other forms of nonallergic rhinitis and that appears in nasal smears—the eosinophil. However, eosinophils also appear in various forms of allergic rhinitis, and it's not always easy for a physician to distinguish one type of rhinitis from the other. Symptoms are similar to those of allergic rhinitis, including sneezing and runny nose.

Cold Air Rhinitis

Although it's normal to experience some degree of nasal stuffiness and congestion when walking in cold, windy weather, some people are hypersensitive to cold and experience severe nasal reactions, similar to severe allergy symptoms. Although cold air rhinitis does not involve an allergic response (that is, there is no identifiable allergen, and the body's immune system does not appear to gear up to fend off a foreign substance), the resulting symptoms— bouts of sneezing, coughing, severe congestion—can lay the groundwork for a sinus attack.

Hormonal Rhinitis

Fluctuating hormone levels during ovulation or pregnancy or while taking birth control pills can trigger nasal congestion and runny nose. These symptoms may also occur among men and women during sexual excitation.

OTHER ENVIRONMENTAL CAUSES

We've seen that many of the pollutants in the air we breathe can cause allergic rhinitis. But other irritants, such as chlorine and cigarette smoke, can also trigger nasal symptoms and sinus problems, even though they don't cause allergic reactions. Changes in air pressure during diving or flying, and the dry air produced by air-conditioning and heating units, can make the sinuses more vulnerable to infection by viruses and bacteria.

Swimming and Diving

Swimming pools treated with chlorine may lead to sinus attacks because chlorine can irritate the lining of the nose and sinuses.

Scuba divers often experience congestion and infection when water contaminated with bacteria is forced into the sinuses from the nasal passages.

Air Travel

Frequent changes in air pressure during landing and take-off can trigger sinusitis in people who regularly travel by air. (Sinusitis is believed to be the single most common occupation-related disorder among flight attendants.)

If you travel by air while suffering from an upper respiratory infection or allergic rhinitis, your risk of having a sinus attack increases: Pressure on swollen tissues surrounding the sinuses produced during a plane's ascent or descent can cause these tissues to swell further, blocking the sinus ostia.

Cigarette Smoke

In addition to its well-publicized health hazards, smoking can also increase your risk of developing sinusitis. There are literally hundreds of potent irritants in cigarette smoke, any one of which can cause an adverse or allergic reaction that subsequently triggers sinusitis. Cigarette smoke also harms cilia—the tiny hairlike projections in the mucous membranes that are responsible for rhythmically moving mucus out of the nose and sinuses—by slowing them down and preventing them from effectively clearing bacteria and debris out of the respiratory system. Passive cigarette smoke, especially when inhaled by children, carries similar risks (see Chapter 7).

"Forced Air" Heating Systems

Home or office heating systems that force warm air into a room dry out the nose and interfere with its ability to produce mucus. Also, because this type of system uses fans that blow dust-laden warm air around the room, it gives the nose and sinuses more debris to filter, while spreading airborne allergens.

Wood-Burning Stoves

Wood-burning stoves are a source of environmental irritants such as fumes, chemicals released from substances used to promote burning, and chemical compounds released from the burning wood itself—all of which can trigger sinusitis. Wood-burning stoves also dry the air, causing a decrease in the amount of mucus produced to trap debris.

NASAL OBSTRUCTION

Any malformation or deviation in the inner structure of the nose or sinuses can block or partially block the sinus ostia, preventing proper drainage of the sinuses and laying the groundwork for sinusitis. Structural problems in the nasal area can occur as a result of injury, illness, or congenital (present at birth) abnormalities.

Nasal Polyps

Polyps are balloonlike growths on the mucous membrane of the nose, usually caused by chronic inflammation. Polyps can cause congestion, loss of smell, and blockage of the sinus ostia. They usually develop in people between the ages of 20 and 40 and are about twice as common in men as in women.

Deviated Septum

The *septum* is the wall that separates the inside of your nose into a right side and a left side. If that wall is crooked (deviated), the sinus ostia may be partially blocked on one side.

Foreign Bodies

Foreign body is a term used to describe anything that is pushed into the nose and left there. Children are more apt to place an object in the nose than adults (see Chapter 7); however, it is possible, for example, to place a bit of packing in the nose to stop a nosebleed—and forget to remove it. A foreign body can cause inflammation and possible infection in the area of the nose where it is lodged, as well as sinusitis.

Tumor

A benign or malignant (cancerous) tumor can cause nasal obstruction and lead to sinusitis. If you have a tumor in the nose, it blocks the nasal passage/sinus opening.

DENTAL PROBLEMS

Because the roots of the upper teeth are located close to the maxillary sinuses, infections in these roots can extend into the sinus cavity and cause sinusitis. Conversely, sinusitis can sometimes cause pain in the teeth area. A diagnostic examination by your dentist or other specialist may be needed to differentiate between the two conditions (see Chapter 3).

Other conditions affecting the teeth that can cause sinus problems include minor trauma or injury (e.g., chipping a tooth), extensive dental work, or a tooth extraction.

SYSTEMIC PROBLEMS AND
CONGENITAL DISORDERS

Diseases and disorders that affect the immune system and the respiratory system can cause sinusitis. Congenital disorders that appear in childhood, such as cleft palate, choanal atresia, pharyngeal stenosis, immotile cilia syndrome, and cystic fibrosis, are discussed in Chapter 7.

Immune Deficiency

Nasal symptoms predisposing to sinusitis, such as congestion and swollen mucous membranes, can occur as a complication of virtually any immune system disorder—whether caused by a virus such as human immunodeficiency virus (HIV), which causes AIDS; medical treatment such as chemotherapy; or a rheumatologic disorder such as connective tissue disease.

Aspirin Sensitivity

People who have a combination of medical and nasal problems (e.g., bronchial asthma, polyps, and chronic sinusitis) may develop a sensitivity to aspirin. When this happens, they experience a severe reaction to aspirin, which can include exacerbated sinusitis symptoms, hives, or an asthma attack. Worse, they may develop *anaphylaxis*—a very severe and occasionally fatal systemic reaction.

Bronchiectasis

Bronchiectasis is a disorder in which the *bronchi*—the passageways that carry air to and within the lungs—become infected and inflamed. This chronic disorder can lead to persistent coughing, pus secretion, and destruction of the cilia (and hence sinusitis) throughout the respiratory tract. Bronchiectasis is a relatively uncommon disorder that may result from an allergy, pneumonia, influenza, tuberculosis, or other disease that affects the respiratory system.

SINUSITIS AND ASTHMA

The relationship between sinusitis and asthma has been studied extensively over the past few years. Most researchers agree that the two disorders are very closely related—by some estimates, as many as 60 percent of people with asthma also have sinusitis. It's not known as yet whether sinusitis and asthma occur together so often because the two are really manifestations of the same underlying disorder, whether asthma lays the groundwork for sinusitis, or whether—and this hypothesis appears increasingly likely—sinusitis actually plays a role in causing asthma.

One reason why accurate diagnosis and prompt treatment of sinusitis are so important relates to its role in asthma. Many people have experienced substantial relief from asthma after proper medical treatment of sinusitis. Since asthma is a debilitating and potentially life-threatening disorder, reducing its severity by treating underlying sinusitis is an important health-promoting step.

THE ROLE OF STRESS

The role of stress in sinusitis is controversial. Some clinicians claim stress plays no role in the disorder; others are convinced that stress is an important contributor to sinus attacks because it may weaken the immune system, making you more vulnerable to a sinus attack. The best way for you to determine whether stress affects your sinuses is to try relaxation techniques such as those described in Chapter 5. If you feel better and experience some relief from your sinusitis, then it is possible that stressful situations aggravate your sinus condition.

IMPORTANT POINTS ABOUT THE CAUSES OF SINUSITIS

- Many medical and environmental conditions can predispose you to sinusitis.

- Medical conditions that contribute to sinusitis include upper respiratory tract infections, allergies, systemic diseases, asthma, hormonal rhinitis, dental problems, and structural problems in the nose.

- Other conditions that can trigger sinusitis include overuse of nasal sprays, exposure to polluted water, air travel, weather changes, and irritants in the environment.

- The close association between sinusitis and asthma is one reason why promptly diagnosing and treating sinusitis is so important. Recent studies have shown that treating sinusitis can provide significant relief from asthma.

- The role of stress in triggering sinusitis is controversial. To help determine whether stress exacerbates your sinusitis symptoms, try relaxation techniques to see whether your symptoms improve.

THREE

DIAGNOSING SINUSITIS

Runny nose, postnasal drip, congestion, pressure in the cheeks and over the eyes, sore throat, bad breath—all these symptoms are common in sinusitis. But as we've seen in the previous chapter, they can also result from a cold, allergy, or some other disorder. Such symptoms aren't specific enough for your doctor to make a diagnosis of sinusitis based on symptomatology alone.

As a first step in making a diagnosis, your doctor must do a physical examination and take a complete medical history. Then he or she must determine whether your sinuses are inflamed or infected. If sinus disease is found, the cause must also be determined in order for proper treatment (described in the next two chapters) to begin.

In this chapter, we'll tell you how to select a physician who is knowledgeable in sinus disease, and what your physician will look for to make a diagnosis. We'll also review the imaging techniques that allow your physician to obtain views of the sinuses, including transillumination, X rays, computed tomography (CT) scan, magnetic resonance imaging (MRI), and ultrasound. The use of endoscopy for viewing the ostiomeatal complex—the area where the sinuses drain into the nose and throat—is also covered. Finally, you'll learn which additional tests may be needed if your doctor suspects that sinusitis is associated with other disorders such as allergies or asthma.

SELECTING A PHYSICIAN

Who can accurately diagnose sinusitis, including the disease or disorder that is causing it? Who can then be counted on to prescribe the appropriate medicine and follow up on your progress? Ideally, this person would be your present physician—a general practitioner or internist who knows you and your medical history, who is knowledgeable about you as a person and as a patient, and who keeps current on diagnostic techniques and treatment of sinusitis. If you do have such a physician, this is the first person you should see if you suspect you are suffering from sinusitis.

It's very possible that you don't now have such a doctor, however. Years ago, many families had a family physician who followed them over many years, handling the common disorders that didn't necessarily require special skills and training to diagnose and treat. But the dramatic changes that have taken place in our health care system in recent years have changed this situation for many people. Today, you may belong to a managed care system or have a health care plan that permits you to choose from among a small pool of member physicians, rather than selecting from among all physicians. If this is the case for you, then your choices may be limited. Nevertheless, most health care plans do permit you at least some choice. So if you don't feel comfortable with your present physician, you should exercise your right to make other choices.

Following are some tips for finding the physician who is right for you and who can treat your sinusitis or refer you to an appropriate specialist.

General Practitioner or Specialist?

If you suspect you have sinusitis, a general practitioner may be able to diagnose and treat you directly, especially if your sinus symptoms are not too severe and appear to result from a cold or bout with the flu, rather than from an allergy, underlying disease, or structural problem in the nose. He or she should also be aware of the latest innovations in diagnosis and treatment of sinusitis, which are covered in this book.

If your sinus symptoms are severe and recurring, or if they appear to be caused by some underlying problem, your physician will probably refer you to a specialist, usually an *otolaryngologist* or *otorhinolaryngologist*—better known as an ear, nose, and throat doctor. If an allergy is suspected, you may be referred to an *allergist* or *immunologist*.

Specialists may perform additional diagnostic tests before prescribing medicine for sinusitis and any underlying disorder. If surgery seems indicated, your options should also be discussed with you (see Chapter 6 for details about sinus surgery).

What to Look for in a Physician: A Checklist

A good physician—whether a general practitioner or a specialist—is someone who provides you with information in a forthright way, treats you with respect and concern, and has an office staff that is efficient and friendly. It makes good sense to "doctor shop" before you have a problem that demands urgent treatment. This checklist provides you with questions to ask yourself during the selection process.

Does this doctor:

____ Communicate with me in a way I can understand, without being condescending? Allow me to express fears about my symptoms or certain forms of treatment? Give me real information about my condition instead of a simple pat on the back and reassurance?

____ Seem knowledgeable about sinusitis, including preventive strategies, and the latest diagnostic and treatment techniques described in this book?

____ Explain medical tests and procedures before performing them? Discuss possible side effects or complications?

____ Take time to answer all my questions without rushing me?

____ Talk with me as a person before beginning the examination? Treat me courteously and with respect?

____ Behave in an authoritarian way? Have an easygoing manner?

_____ Seem comfortable with the idea of my getting a second opinion? Seem threatened and defensive?

_____ Have a staff that is efficient and friendly?

_____ Have regular office hours during the day, evenings, and on weekends? Have a backup physician when he or she is not available?

_____ Regularly keep to the appointment schedule instead of keeping me waiting for long periods in the waiting room?

_____ Permit me to pay over time when visits aren't covered by insurance?

_____ Permit me to pay by check or credit card?

When seeking a new physician, compile a list of doctors whose work is praised by people you respect—friends, family members, community leaders, other health care workers, other physician specialists. You may also consult the *Dictionary of Medical Specialists.*

Next, set up consultation appointments with each prospective physician. Be prepared to pay a fee, usually equal to the fee of a standard office visit. When setting the consultation appointment, get as much information as you can about how the doctor runs the practice, including office hours, waiting time for appointments, and payment schedule. In addition to getting helpful information, asking questions permits you to assess the cordiality and professionalism of the office staff.

MAKING AN INITIAL DIAGNOSIS

In many cases, a skilled physician can make a diagnosis of sinusitis based on your symptoms, your medical history, and a physical examination, without taking additional tests. This is especially true if your sinus symptoms are not very severe, and no serious complications are suspected. Under these circumstances, your physician may prescribe a course of antibiotics for three weeks, possibly along with medication to relieve symptoms, as described in the next chapter.

You would be instructed to schedule another visit after completing the antibiotics. If your sinuses appear clear and you are symptom free, you need go no further unless symptoms begin again shortly afterward. If your sinusitis has not cleared up after treatment, then additional tests, such as X rays, CT scan, and endoscopy—using a tube with a tiny microscope attached to visualize upper nasal passages—may be ordered.

Symptom Review

As we saw in Chapter 1, an acute sinus attack may bring on a wide range of symptoms, including nasal stuffiness and loss of the sense of smell, green or yellow nasal secretions, postnasal drip, bad breath, cough, facial pain, and headache. If an attack is the result of infection, then fever, sore throat, and toothache may also be present. These symptoms, especially on the heels of an upper respiratory tract infection, are clues of a possible sinus infection.

The location of facial pain or headache pain can sometimes provide a starting point for pinpointing the affected sinus. Here's a quick overview of the areas of pain caused by sinusitis:

- *Maxillary sinusitis.* May cause pain over the upper cheeks and teeth.

- *Frontal sinusitis.* May cause pain in the forehead area.

- *Ethmoid sinusitis.* May cause pain around the eyes, or you may have a headache.

- *Sphenoid sinusitis.* May cause severe pain behind the eyes, radiating to the back of the neck.

Medical History

A thorough medical history can, of course, determine whether you have had sinus attacks in the past, whether a physician has diagnosed sinusitis, and if so, what course of treatment you followed. This is important for several reasons. If a sinus attack was successfully treated in the past, your present physician should know which medications were effective. On the other hand, if you've had recurring sinus attacks with symptoms that interfere with your ability to work and socialize, then now may be the time for additional tests to determine whether some underlying, untreated disorder such as an allergy or a structural problem in the nose is triggering your sinusitis. If this is your first sinus attack, aggressive medical treatment as described in the next chapter may prevent sinusitis from becoming chronic.

Here are some of the questions you may be asked during the medical history. It's a good idea to come to your initial doctor visit prepared with answers to these questions:

____ When did your symptoms start?

____ Have you had these symptoms before?

____ Did your sinus symptoms begin after a cold or flu?

____ Were you ever treated for sinusitis before? If so, what form of treatment was used?

____ Do you have any allergies?

____ Does anyone in your family have allergies or sinus problems?

____ Have you experienced any recent stress?

____ Has a physician ever told you that you have a deviated septum, polyps, or other problems in your nose? If so, what was the advice for treating the problem?

____ Are your present symptoms worse than usual, or have you been experiencing them more frequently than usual?

____ Do you have a fever now, and did you have one in the past with these symptoms?

____ Do you have other symptoms that are not related to your sinuses, such as unusual pain, rashes, dizziness, or fatigue?

Physical Examination

After taking your medical history, your doctor should give you a complete physical examination. The examination is likely to vary somewhat from physician to physician and will also vary by specialty—for example, whether you are seeing a general practitioner or a specialist such as an ear, nose, and throat doctor. The examination is also likely to be more detailed if you are experiencing systemic symptoms, such as fever and unusual pain, in addition to nasal and sinus symptoms.

The basics would include taking your temperature if you have had a fever; taking your blood pressure; listening to your heart and lungs; examining your eyes; examining your ears; examining your throat; examining your maxillary and frontal sinuses with a light (see "Transillumination," page 47); and examining the lymph nodes in your neck and under your arms if a systemic infection is suspected.

If your physical examination reveals no other problems, and your medical history is typical of someone with sinusitis, your physician will probably make that diagnosis. However, if you are experiencing very severe or frequent symptoms, or if your sinus symptoms appear to be triggered in connection with an allergy or asthma, then additional tests may be performed to make sure your treatment plan is a complete one. These tests may include more extensive diagnostic imaging of the sinuses and tests for allergy or asthma.

DIAGNOSTIC IMAGING OF THE SINUSES

Common diagnostic imaging tests for sinusitis include transillumination, sinus X rays, and CT scan. MRI is used only in severe disease to rule out chronic fungal sinusitis or a tumor. Ultrasound tests are not recommended. Endoscopy may be used to visualize a common area of sinus blockage, the ostiomeatal complex.

Transillumination

In this procedure, the physician shines a light across the maxillary or frontal sinuses and sees how much light is transmitted through the palate and back into the mouth. If much of the light is blocked (e.g., doesn't shine through), then the sinus is thought to be clogged.

As a diagnostic technique for sinusitis, transillumination has several drawbacks. Since there are no standards for the amount of light that should be reflected (this would be difficult to quantify and varies from person to person), physicians must decide on their own if the amount of light reflected is normal or abnormal. Studies have shown tremendous variability from physician to physician in diagnosing sinus disease from transillumination —meaning that the technique is not accurate except in cases where there is gross, unmistakable blockage of a sinus. Another drawback is that the ethmoid and sphenoid sinuses cannot be viewed with transillumination, so disease cannot be detected in these areas.

However, if your symptoms appear to be due to infection or inflammation of the maxillary or frontal sinuses, transillumination may be used as part of the initial overall physical examination to help confirm a diagnosis.

X Rays

Taking X rays of the sinuses—technically known as *plain radiography*—has long been accepted as the standard test for diagnosing sinus disease. In the past couple of years, however, X rays have been supplanted by CT, described on page 49, as the diagnostic test of choice. Nevertheless, many physicians continue to use X rays to help pinpoint sinus disease, especially if they suspect the problem is in the frontal or maxillary sinuses.

Initially, your physician takes two views of your sinuses, one through your face (Caldwell view) and the other through your chin (Waters view). If the sphenoid sinuses are thought to be involved, then an additional view (lateral view) of these sinuses will be taken. These views may indicate clogging of the sinuses, either by fluid or diseased tissue.

Sinus X rays also suffer from interpretation variability due to differences in perception by physicians, as well as variations in the quality of the radiographs. In addition, abnormal sinus images may occur in people who have no sinus symptoms. For these reasons, sinus X rays alone cannot diagnose sinus disease, nor can they necessarily determine the cause of sinus disease if it does exist. Although an X ray may be able to pick up a structural abnormality, it cannot tell the physician whether sinusitis is related to allergy or to some other disorder; this would have to be determined during the medical history and physical examination or through additional tests.

Computed Tomography

CT scan has recently become the test of choice for diagnosing sinusitis and pinpointing the area and type of damage that is causing symptoms. Unlike standard sinus X rays, a CT screen can also visualize the ethmoid sinuses, a frequent location of inflammation or infection.

A typical CT screen of the sinuses involves four *coronal,* or vertical, views of the head (most CT scans of the head are *axial,* or horizontal). Special settings on the CT scanner, called *bone window settings,* are used to visualize the soft tissue lining the sinuses. A CT screen is often sufficient to diagnose sinusitis and determine the location of inflamed or diseased tissue—though again, as for X rays, additional tests may be needed if the underlying cause of sinusitis is thought to be allergy or systemic illness.

Magnetic Resonance Imaging

MRI is not indicated as a test for sinusitis except in rare cases when an individual has a severe systemic disease such as cancer or chronic fungal sinusitis is suspected. MRI is not considered useful or necessary in diagnosing sinusitis caused by inflammation or infection.

Ultrasound

Ultrasound—the use of sound waves emitted by a device called a *transducer,* which is placed on the skin over the sinus area or other part of the body to be viewed—has fallen into disfavor as a test for sinusitis. This technique cannot detect thickening of the mucosal lining of the maxillary sinuses—a common sinusitis symptom; nor can it detect ethmoid sinus disease. Ultrasound should not be ordered for diagnosing sinusitis.

Endoscopy

Using an *endoscope*—a tube that acts like a tiny telescope —permits a detailed examination of the area in which the sinuses drain into the nose and throat, known as the osti-omeatal complex.

Two types of endoscopes can be used. The *flexible endoscope* is especially useful in revealing polyps and other structural abnormalities in these areas. To use the flexible endoscope, the physician applies a topical anesthetic before inserting the instrument into your nose.

The *rigid endoscope,* which is also used in sinus surgery (see Chapter 6), can be used to visualize the maxillary sinus ostia, which can't be seen with the flexible endoscope. A larger amount of topical anesthesia is applied before the physician inserts the rigid endoscope.

Endoscopy is used when a person has unusual and severe sinus symptoms that can't be effectively treated with medication. Because a good deal of technical skill is required to use the endoscope and accurately interpret what is viewed, this technique should only be used by a physician with extensive training and experience. See Chapter 3 for tips on selecting an appropriate physician, and Chapter 6 for selecting a physician skilled in endoscopy.

OTHER DIAGNOSTIC TESTS

Certain additional tests may be helpful in determining the presence and possible cause of sinusitis. Antral puncture and nasal smears may be useful in confirming a diagnosis of sinusitis in conjunction with one or more of the tests described above. Allergy tests can be useful in identifying a specific allergy in which nasal symptoms contribute to sinusitis. An individual who suffers from asthma should undergo diagnostic tests for sinusitis because sinusitis is a common asthma trigger.

Antral Puncture

Antral puncture (*antrum* = "cavity" or "chamber") is usually performed by a specialist in ear, nose, and throat disorders (see Chapters 3 and 6 for advice on selecting a sinus specialist). Antral puncture is done in severe or prolonged cases of sinusitis when standard medical treatment fails or your symptoms persist despite taking a standard course of medication.

In this procedure, the physician inserts a needle-type tool into the maxillary sinuses through the nose or through the lip. Fluid from the sinus is aspirated out and cultured to determine the cause of infection.

Sometimes, a sinus specialist will also irrigate the maxillary sinuses when doing antral puncture, to flush out fluid and tissue debris that may be clogging the sinuses. This technique, known as *therapeutic lavage,* may be helpful in clearing the maxillary sinuses and relieving symptoms.

Nasal Smear

A nasal smear—looking at tissue from the nose under a microscope—can be used to detect the presence of a type of white blood cell called an *eosinophil.* Since eosinophils play a role in the body's immune responses, their presence in the nose may indicate allergic rhinitis or asthma.

However, eosinophils may also be present in the nose of people who don't have nasal allergies or asthma (see "Nonallergic, Eosinophilic Rhinitis," page 29), so this test cannot be used on its own to determine the cause of sinusitis. But it can help confirm a diagnosis in combination with a physical examination and medical history, or it can point to the need for allergy testing.

Allergy Tests

As we saw in Chapters 1 and 2, sinusitis frequently arises as a complication of nasal congestion caused by allergic rhinitis. If your sinusitis is triggered by allergy symptoms, it's important to treat both sinusitis and the allergy for maximum symptom relief.

Skin Testing for Allergens.   Skin testing is the diagnostic test of choice for discovering whether a person has allergic rhinitis and, if so, which among the common allergens may be causing an allergic reaction. A blood test known as the *radioallergosorbent test* (*RAST*) may also be used. However, according to experts at the National Jewish Center for Immunology and Respiratory Medicine, skin testing is usually sufficient to determine allergy.

There are two types of skin-testing techniques. In one method, an extract of a suspected allergen is injected into the surface layer of the skin, which raises a small bubble on the skin. In the second method, known as the *skin prick method,* a drop of extract is introduced into a deeper layer of the skin using a sharp instrument, causing a small break in the skin.

Both skin tests provide immediate results and are simple to perform and relatively inexpensive. The injection method is more sensitive in identifying allergens, but it's so sensitive that it sometimes identifies insignificant allergens that aren't causing symptoms. The skin prick method is simpler and enables the clinician to test many allergens in one session.

Skin testing for allergens is not 100 percent accurate; results may vary from person to person, and improper use of the technique may affect the findings. However, when used in combination with a complete medical history, skin tests can be very effective in helping to determine whether you are allergic, and if so, to which allergens.

Food Allergy Tests.   Skin testing with food substances may be used to facilitate the diagnosis of food sensitivity. A negative food skin test is believed to be a fairly accurate gauge of whether foods are causing an adverse immune reaction in an individual. Conversely, a positive food skin test can be used as a guide for deciding which foods can be used in a test called a *double-blind food challenge*.

In the double-blind food challenge, suspect foods and neutral, or *placebo,* foods are put into opaque capsules or puddings, then swallowed by the person being tested.

Neither the patient nor the physician knows which capsules or puddings contain the suspect food and which ones contain the placebo. If a person has an allergic reaction to a suspect food under these conditions, a cause-and-effect relationship between the food and the reaction may be established.

If a particular food is already suspected of causing allergic symptoms, your physician may simply ask you to avoid that food for a period of several weeks to see whether you continue to have symptoms. This is called an *elimination diet*.

Pet Allergy Test.   If you think you are allergic to a pet, your physician may recommend doing a *pet challenge*. This involves removing the pet from your home for a period of time to see whether you continue to have symptoms. Since this can be very difficult to do, some people prefer to follow strategies such as those outlined in Chapter 5 (see "Coping with Pets," page 86) to help relieve symptoms.

Diagnosing Nonallergic Causes of Sinusitis

There are no diagnostic tests for the various forms of nonallergic rhinitis and environmentally caused symptoms. That's why a complete medical history is so important. Your history can help reveal sensitivities to weather, pollutants, hormones, and other factors that may trigger sinus symptoms.

Sometimes keeping a diary for a month or so, noting when symptoms occur and what seems to be happening prior to symptoms (e.g., high humidity, air travel, swimming, exposure to cigarette smoke, menstrual cycle changes), can also be helpful. Bring this diary with you to discuss during your doctor visit.

Diagnosing Structural Problems

Structural problems in the nose such as nasal polyps or a deviated septum may be diagnosed during sinus imaging, using the techniques described above. Foreign bodies and tumors may also be identified through this process.

Diagnosing Dental Problems

A dental problem that is triggering sinus symptoms is likely to be identified by your dentist. However, it may also be diagnosed by your physician or specialist during physical examination and discussion of your symptoms.

Diagnosing Systemic Illness

It is beyond the scope of this book to cover the tests used to diagnose systemic disorders and diseases such as immune deficiency and bronchial problems that can predispose a person to sinusitis. In most cases, these illnesses are diagnosed before sinusitis symptoms appear. Once symptoms suggestive of sinusitis occur, your physician's responsibility is to accurately diagnose sinus disease and prescribe treatment that doesn't conflict with any medicines being taken for the underlying illness.

Sinus Tests and Asthma

As we learned in Chapter 2, recent studies have revealed a close relationship between sinusitis and asthma. Many physicians now believe that sinusitis is an important asthma trigger; by treating sinusitis, asthma symptoms and the frequency of asthma attacks may be significantly reduced. For this reason, people with asthma that is not effectively controlled should have a diagnostic CT screen or sinus X ray to determine whether their sinuses are inflamed or infected.

If an individual with asthma also has sinusitis, prompt medical treatment of sinusitis, as described in Chapter 4, and ongoing use of appropriate nonmedical strategies such as environmental control and stress reduction, as described in Chapter 5, can be very beneficial.

IMPORTANT POINTS ABOUT
DIAGNOSING SINUSITIS

- Sinusitis symptoms aren't specific enough to make a diagnosis based on symptomatology alone. A physician must look inside your sinuses to determine whether they are inflamed or infected. Additional tests may be ordered to determine the cause of sinusitis.

- It's important to select a physician who is knowledgeable in the latest techniques for diagnosing and treating sinusitis and its causes. This physician may be a general practitioner or a specialist.

- A diagnosis of sinusitis should be made after a complete physical examination, complete medical history, assessment of your symptoms, and visualization of your sinuses.

- Various techniques are used to visualize the sinuses. A CT scan has become the screening test of choice. Additional tests may be ordered when sinusitis symptoms are very severe or don't respond to medical treatment.

- Once a diagnosis of sinusitis is confirmed, additional tests—particularly allergy tests—may be ordered to determine the underlying cause. Sometimes a careful review of your medical history and symptoms is all that is needed to identify the cause of your sinus symptoms.

- People with asthma should undergo sinus visualization tests because sinusitis—even with very mild symptoms—can trigger asthma attacks.

FOUR

MEDICAL TREATMENT FOR SINUSITIS AND RELATED DISORDERS

The goals of medical treatment for sinusitis are threefold:

- To control infection

- To reduce swelling of the mucous membranes in the nose and sinuses, thereby clearing the sinus ostia

- To ensure that the sinuses remain unclogged and infection free for as long as possible

To accomplish these goals, antibiotics are prescribed to control infection; decongestants may be prescribed to reduce mucosal swelling and facilitate drainage; topical corticosteroids may be used to reduce or prevent inflammation; an expectorant may help you get rid of excess phlegm or mucus; and analgesics may be used to reduce head and facial swelling. We'll look at these medicines in detail in the next sections of this chapter.

Any condition that contributes to sinusitis—allergy, asthma, systemic illness, dental problems, or anatomic abnormality—must also be treated to prevent recurrent sinus attacks. An overview of the medical treatment for these conditions is also described below.

Life-style habits such as cigarette smoking may also need to be changed if you want to experience relief from sinusitis over the long term. These changes are described in Chapter 5, "Nonmedical Techniques."

Your personal treatment plan will depend on several factors, including the severity of your sinus disease, the condition that is causing sinusitis, your medical history (including allergies and sensitivities), and your life-style. Very often, effective treatment includes the use of non-medical strategies at the same time that you are taking medication.

Your physician's knowledge of sinus disease also influences which medicines are prescribed and for how long. It's very important to be treated by a physician who is knowledgeable about sinusitis and aware of current thinking in the diagnosis and treatment of sinus disease (see Chapter 3 for advice on choosing a physician).

Remember that *all* medicines—whether available by prescription or over the counter—can cause side effects in susceptible individuals. Always discuss possible side effects with your physician and pharmacist. If you are taking medication for another condition (anything from antacids to medicine for a serious illness such as heart disease), tell your physician and pharmacist in order to avoid the possibility of harmful interactions among the various drugs. Also find out whether you should take medicine before or after a meal, and the time interval between doses, since these factors can affect a drug's effectiveness. At the end of this chapter, we'll look at how to select a pharmacist who can help coordinate your medications and give you necessary information about prescription and over-the-counter drugs.

Now let's take a closer look at medical treatment for sinusitis in adults. The diagnosis and treatment of sinusitis in children is covered in Chapter 7.

MEDICATIONS THAT TREAT SINUSITIS

Antibiotics are the mainstay of treatment for an active sinus infection. Once the proper antibiotic has been selected, additional medicines may be used to alleviate or prevent blockage of the sinuses. These include decongestants, topical corticosteroids, mucoevacuants, and analgesics. Antihistamines should not be used unless sinusitis is caused by an allergy, since they tend to dry out the sinuses and inhibit the normal production and flow of mucus.

Antibiotics

An active sinus infection should be treated with a *broad-spectrum antibiotic* (broad-spectrum antibiotics kill a wide range of microorganisms) for a minimum of three weeks. Shorter treatment courses (one or two weeks of medicine) may not be sufficient to completely sterilize the sinuses and render them free of infection.

The antibiotics of choice are amoxicillin and ampicillin. Other first-line broad-spectrum antibiotics include amoxicillin with clavulanic acid and cefaclor. These antibiotics are *not* for you if you have a penicillin allergy or sensitivity, however, because ampicillin and amoxicillin are in the penicillin family, and cefaclor may trigger an allergic response in people who are sensitive to penicillin. *Always* tell your physician in advance if you are sensitive or allergic to penicillin. Trimethoprim/sulfamethoxazole is an alternative antibiotic for people who cannot take these medicines.

Antibiotics can cause a wide range of side effects in susceptible individuals. Among the most common are abdominal upset, diarrhea, and skin rash. Antibiotics can also interact with other medications you may be taking, reducing their effect or affecting dosing requirements. Always tell your physician if you are taking any type of medicine on a regular basis, be it a prescription or over-the-counter product. This may affect the selection of an appropriate antibiotic to treat sinusitis.

Decongestants

Decongestants shrink swollen nasal membranes, thereby helping to open the sinus ostia. This promotes the free flow of air through the nose and sinuses, reducing the chance of an infection developing in blocked sinus cavities. Decongestants also relieve the clogged-up feeling often associated with sinusitis.

Decongestants come in two forms: *topical* (nasal sprays or drops) and *systemic* (tablets, liquids, or capsules taken by mouth).

Topical Decongestants. Topical decongestants provide relief within a few minutes because they go right to work on the nose. However, they have a major disadvantage in that they should not be used for more than three days at a time. If used for longer than a few days, these preparations can cause "rebound congestion," sometimes making symptoms even worse than before the medication was started (see "Rhinitis Medicamentosa," page 28, and below). It's best to use topical decongestants for quick, temporary relief of particularly acute symptoms.

Different brands of topical decongestants have different active ingredients, which include *phenylephrine, ephedrine, naphazoline, oxymetazoline,* and *xylometazoline.* If you find that one brand of decongestant is not effective for you, check the label for its active ingredient. Then look for another brand that has a different active ingredient to see whether it works better.

Read the label carefully to make sure you understand dosing requirements (the number of sprays or drops you should use and how often to medicate). Also be aware of possible side effects and discuss these with your physician and pharmacist. Irritation of the lining of the nose and a burning sensation inside the nose are the most common side effects of topical decongestants. However, because some of the medicine is absorbed through the nose into the bloodstream, you may also experience some of the systemic side effects associated with systemic decongestants, described below.

Systemic Decongestants. Systemic decongestants are taken by mouth. They take longer to work than topical decongestants because they must be absorbed by the blood and then carried by circulation to the nose. Because they travel through the body before reaching the nose, systemic decongestants can be absorbed by tissues other than the nose as well. This is why you may experience more side effects with a systemic decongestant than you would with a topical decongestant. An advantage of systemic decongestants is that they do not cause rebound congestion, so they can be taken over long periods of time.

There is a wide variety of systemic decongestants on your pharmacy shelf, with different strengths and dosing requirements. However, the active ingredients in these products are the same: *pseudoephedrine, phenylpropanolamine, phenylephrine,* or a combination of these decongestants. The decision of which to use will be determined by how much medicine you need to take on a daily basis, as well as which mode of dosing (pill or liquid, timed-released or regular) you prefer.

The dosage of active medication required for effectiveness is much higher in systemic decongestants than in topical decongestants, which means side effects of the systemic products are more common and potentially more severe. Pregnant and lactating women and people with heart disease, high blood pressure, enlarged prostate, diabetes, and other diseases and disorders should take systemic decongestants only under the advice and guidance of a physician.

Potential side effects of these medications include drowsiness, nervousness, gastrointestinal upset, insomnia, vision problems, and mood disturbances. You may need to experiment among the different products available to see which provide you with relief while producing the fewest possible side effects.

Mucoevacuants

When sinusitis causes mucus to become very thick, a mucoevacuant, also known as an *expectorant,* may be prescribed to help you get rid of excess phlegm and mucus from the nose, chest, and throat. The most common is *guaifenesin,* which is also an ingredient in many combination over-the-counter pills that contain both a decongestant and an expectorant.

Topical Corticosteroids

When sinusitis is associated with allergic rhinitis or nasal polyps, corticosteroid synthetic hormone nasal sprays may be used to reduce nasal inflammation, thereby facilitating opening of the sinus ostia. Since an inflamed nose is often runny, stuffy, itchy, and twitchy, corticosteroid nasal sprays can reduce or eliminate these symptoms.

Topical corticosteroids generally take up to three weeks to become effective. They should be used regularly, according to the dosing recommendations on the label.

Unlike oral and injectable corticosteroids, which are associated with severe side effects, the nasal corticosteroid sprays generally produce very mild side effects. An exception is dexamethasone, the first corticosteroid spray introduced in this country. Although effective in relieving nasal symptoms, this corticosteroid is very easily absorbed by the body and may cause severe systemic side effects such as increases in blood pressure, puffiness of the face, ulcers, muscle wasting, and osteoporosis. It should not be used over long periods of time.

The newer corticosteroid nasal sprays—with active ingredients *beclomethasone, flunisolide,* or *triamcinolone* —are associated with milder, local side effects such as irritation of the lining of the nose.

Any of the corticosteroid sprays may cause bleeding, ulceration, and possible perforation of the septum. If you experience severe or frequent nosebleeds while using these medications, see your physician immediately.

Analgesics

If your sinusitis symptoms include headache, facial pain, or sore throat, over-the-counter analgesics may be used to relieve pain and reduce inflammation. Products that contain aspirin or ibuprofen relieve pain and may reduce inflammation of the mucous membranes of the nose and sinuses; products that contain acetaminophen relieve pain but do not reduce inflammation.

To avoid the stomach upset that sometimes occurs when you take several aspirins daily, use brands that are "coated." Older adults and others who may be susceptible to gastrointestinal bleeding from aspirin should take an acetaminophen medication instead (remember, acetaminophen won't relieve inflammation).

As we saw in Chapter 2, some people who have chronic medical problems as well as nasal and sinus problems may develop a sensitivity to aspirin and should avoid taking it.

Avoiding Antihistamines

The only time antihistamines should be used in sinusitis is when the condition occurs in association with allergies (see page 70). These medications can dry out the sinuses and interfere with the reestablishment of normal mucous production and flow.

Treating Fungal Sinus Infections

Most sinus infections are caused by bacteria or viruses that grow in the dark, moist environment of the clogged sinuses. However, in rare cases—mostly in individuals whose immune systems are weakened by disease or age— fungal infections occur, causing secretions of very thick mucus. The infected sinus must be thoroughly cleaned and the inner lining scraped with a surgical tool. Then antifungal medication is administered by injection.

MEDICATION FOR CONDITIONS ASSOCIATED WITH SINUSITIS

In addition to treating symptoms of sinusitis, any medical condition that leads to sinusitis should also be treated— otherwise, your sinus attacks are likely to recur. In some cases, treatment for the underlying cause of sinusitis is straightforward. For example, if overuse of a nasal spray causes rebound congestion leading to sinusitis, you must stop using the spray.

In many instances, however, treatment of the disorder

that is causing sinusitis can be complicated, involving different types of medicines and life-style changes. This is often the case when sinusitis is caused by allergies or environmental factors.

When severe or recurring sinusitis symptoms occur as a result of polyps, a structural abnormality in the nose, or an infection that doesn't respond to treatment with antibiotics, surgery may be considered. Sinus surgery is discussed in detail in Chapter 6.

UPPER RESPIRATORY TRACT INFECTION

Sinusitis frequently develops after an upper respiratory tract infection such as a cold or flu or after a bacterial infection such as a *Staphylococcus* infection. Your stuffed-up nose blocks the sinuses and prevents them from efficiently sweeping out mucus. The sinuses become a breeding ground for viruses and bacteria that would normally be swept away; and because your resistance is lower during and immediately following an upper respiratory tract infection, you're more vulnerable to these microorganisms than you would be if you were completely healthy.

It's not always possible to prevent an upper respiratory tract infection from affecting the sinuses. However, if you take medicine to reduce nasal swelling and stuffiness, you may avoid clogging the sinuses and setting the stage for a sinus infection.

Following are some of the medicines available to treat upper respiratory tract infections.

Antibiotics

If your respiratory infection is due to a bacterial infection, antibiotics such as those described (see pages 60–1) for the treatment of a bacterial sinus infection may be prescribed. If your respiratory infection is due to a virus, antibiotics won't help and should not be prescribed unless there is evidence of a secondary sinus infection.

Cold Medicines

Cold medicines is a catchall phrase used to describe the wide range of products that offer symptom relief for colds and flu. You may purchase cold medicines that contain decongestants, analgesics, mucoevacuants, antitussives (cough relief ingredients), and various combinations of each.

A rule of thumb to remember when purchasing over-the-counter symptom-relief medicine is to keep it *simple*. Don't pay more, and overload your body with all different types of medicine, unless you know you really need all the ingredients a combination product contains.

If your nose is stuffy, use a decongestant. If you have lots of mucus, try a product that also has a mucoevacuant. For pain relief, you may prefer simple aspirin or acetaminophen on their own. Don't purchase a medicine that contains an antitussive unless you have a severe cough.

Another rule of thumb is to talk to your pharmacist before purchasing an over-the-counter cold medicine. Describe your symptoms and ask for the least expensive, most effective medicine to treat your condition (see the end of this chapter for advice on choosing a pharmacist).

Analgesics

The same guidelines for taking analgesics for sinus symptoms apply to analgesics you may want to take to relieve symptoms of an upper respiratory tract infection.

ALLERGIC RHINITIS

A mainstay of treatment for allergic rhinitis are the antihistamines, which relieve runny nose; sneezing; itching in the nose, throat, or eyes; and postnasal drip. Congestion and stuffiness associated with allergic rhinitis can be relieved by taking a decongestant. A combination product —one that contains an antihistamine and a decongestant —can be helpful if you experience congestion and stuffiness along with one or more of the other symptoms mentioned.

Corticosteroid nasal sprays are used in allergic rhinitis to reduce inflammation of the lining of the nose. Cromolyn sodium, a prescription nasal spray, may be prescribed as a preventive medicine to reduce the likelihood of an allergy attack or to limit its symptoms. Immunotherapy, or "allergy shots," may be recommended to reduce your sensitivity to allergens. Steering clear of environmental allergens (see Chapter 5) can also reduce allergy attacks.

Antibiotics are useless in treating allergies and should

not be prescribed unless the allergy occurs concurrently with an acute bacterial infection.

Antihistamines

Antihistamines are chemical products that work against (*anti*) histamine, a naturally occurring chemical that is released by cells when you come into contact with an allergen.

When tissues that contain receptors for histamine, such as those in the nose, react to the release of histamine, several things happen at once: Blood vessels in the nose become dilated, and the tissues lining the nose swell up. A reaction called *reflex stimulation* also occurs, which causes sneezing and itching. Antistamines counteract this nasal reaction and thus relieve symptoms.

More than a dozen different types of antihistamines are used in over-the-counter and prescription medicines, so finding one that works for you while producing a minimal amount of side effects may take some trial and error. General side effects of antihistamines include drowsiness, irregular heartbeat, abdominal cramps, nausea, constipation, and blood cell irregularities. Some antihistamine products may cause more of certain types of side effects and less of others. Start by asking your physician or pharmacist which antihistamines seem to cause the fewest side effects in people taking them.

Decongestants

The advice given above for taking decongestants to treat sinusitis symptoms also applies for the treatment of congestion associated with allergic rhinitis.

Antihistamine-Decongestant Combinations

These combination products, available over the counter and by prescription, contain both an antihistamine and a decongestant. They're available in liquid, tablets, and sustained-release tablets of varying formulations and potencies. Before purchasing these products, be sure that you do indeed suffer from symptoms that need both types of medications for relief. Remember that sinusitis should not be treated with a combination product unless you also have an allergy.

Side effects of these products are the same as for all antihistamines and decongestants. With combination products, you may experience side effects from the antihistamine in the product but not the decongestant, or vice versa. Or you may experience side effects from both—or neither. Again, trial and error, and consulting in advance with your physician and pharmacist, will help determine which work for you while producing a minimum of side effects.

Corticosteroid Sprays

Corticosteroid sprays can relieve inflammation in allergic rhinitis as well as in sinusitis. See the guidelines above.

Cromolyn Sodium

Unlike antihistamines, decongestants, and corticosteroid sprays, which reduce symptoms after the allergic process has occurred, cromolyn sodium actually blocks certain allergic reactions in the nose from occurring. Cromolyn sodium appears to be effective in preventing runny nose and sneezing but not congestion and stuffiness.

Side effects of cromolyn sodium include sneezing immediately after use, a burning sensation in the nose, a bad taste in the mouth, or increased postnasal drip.

Immunotherapy

Immunotherapy consists of a series of injections of solutions of the allergen or allergens believed to be causing your symptoms (these are identified through a skin or RAST test, described in Chapter 3). By gradually exposing the body to stronger and stronger concentrations of the culprit allergens, you may become "desensitized" to them. In simple terms, this means your body adapts to their presence so they no longer trigger an allergic reaction and allergic symptoms.

The value of immunotherapy in preventing allergic reactions is controversial. According to the National Jewish

Center for Immunology and Respiratory Medicine, immunotherapy has proven effective against the following allergens: grass pollen, ragweed pollen, birch pollen, mountain cedar pollen, house dust, house dust mite, cat and dog dander, and insect venom.

Immunotherapy is specific against only the allergens used in the treatment. So if you happen to be allergic to both ragweed pollen and grass pollen, for example, you must be treated for both; if you are treated for ragweed pollen only, you will continue to experience a reaction to grass pollen.

Immunotherapy may take months or even years to become effective. Because there is a risk of anaphylactic shock (a severe, sometimes fatal, allergic reaction) shortly after an injection, immunotherapy requires careful medical monitoring.

Avoiding Environmental Triggers

The most effective way to avoid allergic rhinitis—and the possibility of developing sinusitis as a consequence of this disorder—is to avoid those substances in the environment that trigger an allergic reaction. Strategies for avoiding environmental exposure to allergens are discussed in the next chapter.

Avoiding Antibiotics

Antibiotics have no effect on allergies and should not be prescribed or taken as a means to prevent or relieve allergy symptoms.

FOOD ALLERGIES

The connection between food allergies and sinusitis is controversial. Strategies to determine whether specific foods cause nasal symptoms (and may therefore lead to sinusitis) are discussed in Chapter 3. Meal-planning strategies to avoid suspect foods may be discussed with a registered dietitian.

NONALLERGIC RHINITIS

Treatment of nonallergic rhinitis usually consists of various combinations of the prescription and over-the-counter medicines described above, as well as avoidance of the substances that precipitate symptoms.

Here is a brief overview of medical treatment strategies for nonallergic rhinitis that predisposes a person to sinusitis.

Eosinophilic, Nonallergic Rhinitis

This disorder, which appears to be triggered by weather and air pressure changes, may respond to treatment with decongestants and topical cromolyn or corticosteroids.

Rhinitis Medicamentosa

Abrupt withdrawal of a nasal decongestant may lead to rebound congestion (see Chapter 2). Nasal or oral corticosteroids may be used to treat congestion during the withdrawal period.

Vasomotor Rhinitis

This condition of unknown origin causes symptoms when you're exposed to irritants in the environment. Decongestants and topical steroids can usually help relieve symptoms.

Cold Air Rhinitis

Avoidance or protection from cold air is the first line of defense against this form of nonallergic rhinitis. You can also try the now-familiar array of medicines that treat allergic rhinitis symptoms, described above.

At this writing, two new nasal sprays (atropine and ipratropium) are awaiting Food and Drug Administration (FDA) approval for treatment of this disorder.

Hormonal Rhinitis

If your sinus symptoms are related to hormones, your best course of action is to plan to treat symptoms at the time of the month that you are affected. If sinusitis is related to birth control pills, consider trying other brands or—if your sinusitis symptoms are severe—stopping birth control pills altogether and using another form of birth control.

OTHER ENVIRONMENTAL CAUSES

No specific medical treatment will reduce your vulnerability to chlorine irritation, dry air or pressure changes during air travel, or dry air produced by air-conditioning and heating systems. As discussed in the next chapter, the most you can do is minimize your exposure to such environmental irritants.

If you smoke cigarettes—a major nonallergic environmental cause of nasal irritation and sinusitis—quit now. A variety of strategies are available to help you, including nicotine patches prescribed by your physician.

NASAL OBSTRUCTIONS

Decongestants and topical corticosteroids can often control nasal polyps. Surgery may be helpful in severe cases; however, polyps tend to reappear after surgery—a fact that should be kept in mind if you're considering this option (see Chapter 6).

A deviated septum can also be straightened by surgery. However, the septum may also move back to its deviated position following surgery.

A foreign body lodged in the nose will need to be removed by your physician. In rare instances, surgery may be required to remove the object.

A tumor in the nose should be biopsied (a small tissue sample is removed and examined under a microscope) to determine whether it is benign or malignant (cancerous). Your physician will discuss treatment options with you, based on the biopsy results.

DENTAL PROBLEMS

If a dental problem is suspected as the cause of sinusitis, you should be referred to your regular dentist or an *endodontist* (a specialist in the treatment of conditions that affect the tooth pulp, root, and surrounding tissues).

SYSTEMIC PROBLEMS

In most cases, systemic problems resulting in a compromised immune system require aggressive medical treatment, which will vary considerably, depending on the disease or disorder. Once the underlying problem is treated, sinusitis may clear up or be significantly improved.

ASTHMA

It is beyond the scope of this book to describe the full course of medical treatment for asthma. However, it is important to note that if your asthma is not effectively controlled, you should also be tested for sinusitis (see Chapter 3).

If sinusitis is diagnosed, an appropriate course of treatment, described above, should be prescribed. Recent studies have shown that when sinusitis symptoms are controlled, the frequency and severity of asthma attacks are reduced.

SELECTING A PHARMACIST

Many people don't realize that a pharmacist, like any other health professional, should be chosen with care. Registered pharmacists have special training and education in pharmaceuticals—prescription and over-the-counter drugs. They are often in the best position to talk with you about potential side effects of medication, possible interactions among various medicines you may be taking, how often to take your medicine, whether to have it before or with meals, and any other issues pertaining to the medicine you may take to treat your sinusitis symptoms. Although these issues should also be discussed with your doctor, the reality is that your physician may not always be aware of all aspects of importance for each and every medication. That is the responsibility of the pharmacist.

Like a good physician, a good pharmacist should be

willing to talk with you about your medicine and respond to your questions and concerns. The pharmacist can also act as a coordinator of your medications, staying alert to possible adverse interactions among them. Many pharmacies today have computerized records for each customer, noting all the medications they are taking (assuming, of course, that you purchase them in the same pharmacy). Some also have special computer software that automatically alerts them to potential adverse drug interactions when an additional medicine is prescribed.

Equally important when it comes to sinusitis, a pharmacist is well versed in over-the-counter medicines. Your pharmacist can help you select appropriate medicines, such as a decongestant, antihistamine, or combination product, to treat your symptoms during times when it may not be necessary to see your physician. He or she can also help you select among various products that may offer the same active ingredients—but at different prices.

When you have a chronic condition such as sinusitis that generally requires you to take some type of medicine over an extended period of time, it's in your best interest to make friends with your pharmacist and make use of his or her specialized knowledge. The way to tell whether a pharmacist will be responsive to your needs is to ask questions and gauge the pharmacist's willingness to respond candidly and helpfully.

Of course, cost of medication is also an important factor. You probably won't want to patronize a pharmacy that consistently offers products at higher prices than other nearby pharmacies. However, once you establish a relationship with a pharmacist where medications are competitively priced, if you happen to see a product advertised for less at a competing pharmacy, you may ask if your pharmacist will meet that price.

IMPORTANT POINTS ABOUT MEDICAL TREATMENT OF SINUSITIS

- The goals of medical treatment for sinusitis are to control infection, reduce swelling of the mucous membranes in the nose and sinuses, and ensure that the sinuses remain unclogged and infection free for as long as possible.

- Antibiotics are prescribed to control infection. Decongestants reduce mucosal swelling. Topical corticosteroids reduce or prevent inflammation. An expectorant helps you get rid of excess phlegm or mucus. Analgesics reduce head and facial swelling.

- Conditions that contribute to sinusitis, such as allergy, asthma, systemic illness, dental problems, or anatomic abnormalities, must also be treated to prevent recurrent sinus attacks.

- Your treatment plan depends on the severity of your sinus disease, the condition that is causing sinusitis, your medical history (including allergies and sensitivities), and your life-style. Effective treatment may include the use of nonmedical strategies at the same time that you are taking medication.

- Select your pharmacist carefully. He or she can discuss potential side effects of medication, possible interactions among various medicines, and other issues relating to taking medication.

• Use the information in this chapter to help you select appropriate medicines for relief of sinusitis symptoms and for conditions that may predispose you to sinus attacks.

FIVE

NONMEDICAL TECHNIQUES

In addition to the medical treatment described in the previous chapter, there are steps you can take on your own to reduce sinusitis symptoms. These strategies should be considered *adjuncts* to medical care—that is, they should be used in addition to, not instead of, a prescribed course of medical treatment.

In this chapter, you'll learn how to keep your home clean and free of dust mites and mold, avoid animal danders, decrease your exposure to pollen, and avoid sinus-irritating heating systems. You'll also learn how to clear the sinuses and facilitate breathing by using steam inhalation, saline nasal sprays, and eating pungent foods.

Staying healthy—following a healthful diet; staying active; using herbs, acupressure, and other stress- and symptom-relieving techniques—can also help you fend off sinus attacks. We'll give you the basics.

It's important to realize that with the probable exception of staying healthy these nonmedical tactics won't work for everyone. For example, keeping your home free of mites, avoiding animal danders, decreasing your exposure to pollen, and eliminating certain foods from your diet are important only if your sinusitis is triggered by allergies or asthma; if you are not allergic or asthmatic, these steps won't help your sinusitis. However, because many cases of sinusitis do occur in conjunction with allergies—and there are so many different types of allergens —it pays to try some of these techniques to see whether they help, even if you don't think allergies play a role in your particular case.

Steam inhalation, saline nasal sprays, and spicy foods can clear your sinuses and provide some relief from symptoms, regardless of the cause. Although these strategies are short-lived—you must keep repeating them to obtain benefits—they begin to work almost immediately and can be very helpful in the short term.

There are no scientifically proven benefits to using herbal preparations and acupressure techniques to treat sinusitis, which is why they should not be used instead of medical treatment—despite claims to the contrary by people who practice them. However, since some people do experience symptom relief with these approaches, it can't hurt to try them in addition to medication or when you don't have an active sinus infection.

Megadoses of vitamins, minerals, or other substances have no proven benefit in treating sinusitis and may, in fact, be harmful to the body. They are not recommended for self-treatment under any circumstances and should only be used if prescribed by your physician to treat a deficiency. Some people believe supplementation with vitamin C reduces symptoms of colds and sinusitis, although scientific studies have yielded mixed results. You may want to discuss this option with your physician.

On the other hand, it does make good sense to follow a

well-balanced diet, get adequate amounts of rest, and reduce the amount of stress in your life as a hedge against
sinus attacks. Overall good health and a strong immune
system can help fend off disease and may also lessen the
severity of sinusitis symptoms.

ENVIRONMENTAL CONTROL

Controlling Dust and Molds

If your sinusitis is associated with allergies or asthma, one
of the first things you should do is reduce the allergens in
the home. Special emphasis should be placed on getting
rid of allergens in the bedroom, where adults spend approximately one third of their time and children one half
of their time, according to the National Jewish Center for
Immunology and Respiratory Medicine.

Although it is impossible to get rid of house dust and
its components entirely, you can reduce the amount in
your home by taking the following steps:

- Avoid wall-to-wall carpeting. Instead, cover your
  hardwood floors with washable throw rugs that have
  a short nap or vinyl covering.

- Use a tank-type vacuum cleaner with strong suction.
  Vacuum at least once weekly. Wear a surgical mask
  while vacuuming and for at least 15 minutes after
  vacuuming to avoid airborne dust particles.

- Avoid upholstered furniture as much as possible, since it gathers dust. Clean whatever upholstered furniture you have frequently. If you are allergic, don't sit or lie on upholstered furniture.

- Enclose mattresses and box springs in soft plastic covers. Use pillows made of polyester; avoid feathers, foam, and kapok.

- Wash all linen in hot water weekly.

- Buy washable, nonallergic stuffed animals for your children.

- Avoid dust collectors such as quilts, comforters, and canopies. If you use these items, wash them frequently in hot water.

To reduce the growth of molds—also powerful allergens—in the dark, damp areas of your home, take the following steps:

- Use a dehumidifier to reduce moisture levels in the bathroom, kitchen, and basement areas.

- Use a disinfectant or liquid bleach at least once monthly to clean bathtubs, shower stalls, and bath curtains.

- Replace damp carpets and carpet pads.

- Remove leaves, grass clippings, moldy firewood, and compost from the outdoor area within 200 feet of your home.

Coping with Pets

If you are highly allergic to your pet's dander and know that your allergic reaction is causing sinusitis as well, then you may have to give the pet away. But if you are only mildly allergic and live in a home with a backyard, it may be sufficient to keep your pet outside, to avoid frequent contact with dander.

If you live in an apartment and are mildly allergic, follow the steps noted above for controlling house dust to keep your apartment as clean and dander free as possible. Consider having your carpets and upholstered furniture professionally cleaned every six months.

Decreasing Pollen Exposure

Airborne pollens are a common source of allergy that can predispose you to sinusitis. Pollens from shrubs and trees often travel many miles, so you must protect yourself not only from vegetation located right outside your home but also from trees and shrubs in the surrounding neighborhood. Also be aware that pets can bring pollen into the house on their fur. Even visitors to your home can carry pollen on their clothing. Although you won't be able to eliminate your exposure to pollen completely, you can reduce your exposure by taking the following steps:

- During pollen season, keep windows shut and use central or room air conditioners that recirculate indoor air. Don't use window fans, since they can blow pollen into the house. Be aware that pollen seasons vary depending on the tree or shrub and your location. Check with your allergist or one of the organizations listed in the "For More Information" section of this book (see page 136) for the pollen seasons in your hometown or city.

- Mow the lawn frequently to prevent a buildup of pollen. Wear a disposable pollen and dust mask to help filter allergens.

Using Air Filtration Systems

The use of indoor air filters to reduce particle concentration levels of pollen and other allergens is controversial. Ask your allergist for his or her recommendation.

Using House Plants

House plants can promote easier breathing at home and in the office by reducing carbon dioxide levels and releasing oxygen into the air. Some research suggests that plants such as aloe vera, spider plants, and English ivy may also reduce levels of formaldehyde and other irritants known to trigger rhinitis in susceptible people.

If mold develops in the soil of a house plant, remove it; like any mold, it may trigger an allergic reaction that can predispose you to a sinus attack.

Avoiding "Forced Air" Heating

Central heating systems that force warm air into a room dry the sinuses and give them more dust particles to filter. Use another system or don't use the fan.

Avoiding Wood-Burning Stoves

Wood-burning stoves are a source of environmental irritants and also dry the air, thereby reducing the amount of mucus produced by the sinuses. They should be avoided by people with sinusitis.

AVOIDING TRIGGER FOODS

As we saw in Chapter 2, the area of food allergies is a controversial one. But if certain foods seem to trigger congestion, regardless of the reason, then you should take steps to avoid these foods. If you are sensitive to a whole class of foods, such as dairy products or wheat, work with an allergist and a registered dietitian to find alternatives you can live with while maintaining a healthy diet.

CLEARING THE SINUSES

Using Steam Inhalation

Warm steam can help clear much of the buildup of stagnant mucus in the sinuses caused by blockage of the sinus ostia. A wide range of steam-making machines is available (one knowledgeable source says prices range anywhere from $16 to $3,500 for a unit!), but you can probably do the job most efficiently (and inexpensively) by re-creating "granny's steam tent": Simply boil water in a kettle, pour it into a basin, put a large towel over your head, and allow the steam to waft up into your nose and sinuses. Since the steam doesn't last very long, be sure to put up a second kettle once you've poured boiling water into the basin. Some people find that adding eucalyptus, pine, or peppermint oil to the steam makes it more effective.

Steam inhalation can be very effective in relieving sinusitis symptoms and can be repeated over and over (take care not to scald yourself in the process, however). If you have an active sinus infection (as opposed to simply having blocked sinuses), then steam inhalation is useful as an adjunct to medical treatment.

Using Saline Irrigation

Saltwater nasal irrigation can also be very effective in opening up the sinus ostia. It washes out excess mucus and bacteria and reduces swelling of the mucus-producing lining of the nose and sinuses.

If you have an acute sinus infection, irrigate your nose at least three or four times daily with one of the methods described below. If you have chronic sinusitis, but no active infection, irrigating your nose at least twice daily with one of these methods, plus using a saline nasal spray (see next section), should help reduce stuffiness and congestion.

To prepare, mix one pint of boiled water with one teaspoon table salt and a pinch of baking soda. Use approximately one cup of solution for each irrigation, one-half cup for each nostril. It's better to boil water and prepare each irrigation separately, rather than permitting the solution to sit around in a container.

Saline irrigation is a somewhat awkward and uncomfortable procedure. But once you get the hang of it, and experience the free, unhampered breathing it produces, you'll probably adapt very quickly to whichever routine you choose.

- *Method one.* Stand over the sink and keep your head upright. Pour saline solution into the palm of your hand and sniff it up your nose, one nostril at a time. Spit the solution out of your mouth and blow your nose very gently afterward.

- *Method two.* Fill a large, all-rubber ear syringe, available at most pharmacies, with saline solution. Lean over the sink and insert the syringe tip just inside one nostril; pinch the other nostril closed. Gently squeeze and release the bulb of the syringe to swish the solution around inside your nose. Release the other nostril. The solution will run out of both nostrils and probably out of your mouth, as well.

- *Method three.* Use the nasal irrigator attachment included with some oral hygiene appliances. Follow instructions and irrigate one nostril at a time, with your mouth open, to allow the fluid to drain out of your mouth or nose.

Other topical nasal medications, in spray or drop form, should be used *after* the saline irrigation.

Using Saline Sprays

Saline nasal sprays help moisturize the nose to relieve stuffiness, although they are not as effective in clearing mucus as saline irrigation. Nevertheless, when you are in situations that don't permit you to immediately irrigate your nose, using a saline spray is a good alternative. Saline nasal sprays can be purchased inexpensively at most pharmacies. They are not addictive and have no known side effects.

Some people choose to make their own spray to carry in a squeeze bottle. If you decide to do this, you must prepare the solution under sterile conditions or the spray may become a source of infection. This means boiling water first, cleaning the container with boiling water, and wearing plastic gloves while making the solution.

Eating Pungent Foods

Like torpedoes aimed at your clogged sinuses, the pungent oils in certain foods shoot right up your nose and clear up stuffiness—for a few minutes, that is. Chomping on foods such as fresh garlic (not capsules), horseradish, and hot peppers will temporarily clear your sinuses, but once the effect wears off, symptoms return as before.

STAYING HEALTHY

A Healthy Diet

Some evidence suggests that a weakened immune system may make you more vulnerable to sinus attacks. So any measures you take to improve nutrition are apt to help reduce the severity of sinusitis and its symptoms, and other health problems as well.

When planning a healthful diet, keep in mind the seven dietary guidelines recommended by the U.S. Department of Agriculture and the U.S. Department of Health and Human Services and endorsed by the nation's leading health organizations:

1. *Maintain a desirable body weight.* If you're overweight, plan to shed pounds sensibly. If you are already at your desirable weight, plan to maintain it by consuming a moderate amount of calories daily and staying physically active (see page 94).

2. *Eat a varied diet.* This is self-explanatory. As we mentioned earlier, if you are sensitive to certain groups of foods, consult with your physician and a registered dietitian or other nutrition expert to select alternatives.

3. *Include a variety of vegetables and fruits in your daily diet.*

4. *Eat high-fiber foods, such as whole grain cereals, legumes, vegetables, and fruit.*

5. *Cut down on total fat intake.*

6. *Limit consumption of alcoholic beverages.* With respect to sinusitis, use your food diary and elimination strategy (see Chapter 3) to determine whether wine or other sulfite-containing beverages trigger sinus symptoms. Be aware that alcohol may also decrease the motion of the cilia, the hairlike projections that keep mucus flowing freely from the sinuses into the nose and throat.

7. *Limit consumption of salt-cured, smoked, and nitrite-preserved foods.*

An eating plan developed in accordance with these guidelines will help keep your energy up and your immune system strong, which, in turn, should enhance your body's ability to fend off sinus attacks (if you have an immune-deficiency disease, you will have to take medication as well). Work with your physician and other health professionals to plan an appropriate diet for you.

Vitamin Supplements

If you want to take a vitamin supplement to ensure that you get all the nutrients needed daily, take an inexpensive, once-daily vitamin and mineral supplement that contains no more than 100 percent of the recommended dietary allowance for these nutrients. Taking megadoses of vitamins—except under a physician's guidance to treat a deficiency—can be harmful.

Physical Activity

There is no question that regular exercise—especially the aerobic type, such as brisk walking, swimming, cycling, dancing, or classes at your gym or health club—improves health overall and can help you maintain a desirable weight. With respect to sinusitis, regular aerobic exercise can help lessen symptoms by increasing the flow of oxygen to all tissues (including the lungs, nose, and the mucus-producing lining of the sinuses), making it easier for you to breathe and reducing fatigue. Exercise is also a stress reliever and therefore can decrease sinus attacks that are brought on or exacerbated by stress (see pages 98–100 for other stress-reducing techniques).

There are certain precautions you should take with respect to physical exercise. First, consult with your physician before embarking on a new exercise program, especially if you also suffer from asthma (in some individuals, vigorous exercise may trigger an asthma attack). Also, be aware of air quality—indoors and outdoors. When selecting an indoor facility, make sure there is adequate ventilation from open windows or an air-conditioning system that recycles indoor air (systems that pull in air from outdoors may trigger allergic reactions in hay fever sufferers); if large floor or ceiling fans are used, make sure the facility is clean and relatively dust free; otherwise, the fans will blow these irritants into the air you're breathing as you work out.

When exercising outdoors, be aware of ozone levels; high ozone levels (above 0.125 parts per million) can trigger allergic rhinitis (see Chapter 2) and subsequent sinus attacks. When ozone levels are high, as they are on sunny days in the downtown area of large cities, you're better off exercising indoors, where ozone levels may be only half of what they are outdoors.

If you enjoy jogging or cycling along main roads, engage in these activities during off-peak hours to limit your exposure to vehicle pollution.

Whether indoors or outdoors, be sure to choose an activity—and preferably more than one, so you can vary your routine—that you truly enjoy. When you really like working out, you're apt to stick with it until it becomes a normal, enjoyable part of your life. At that point, you're no longer exercising simply because it's "good for my sinuses"; you're exercising because it makes you feel good!

Herbal Preparations

In the past few years, plants and herbs have been "rediscovered" as a potential source of healing medicine. Although few medical professionals would recommend using herbal preparations instead of pharmaceutical medicines to fight a sinus infection, they may be used *in addition to* antibiotics and other prescription drugs. If you suffer from sinusitis symptoms but don't have an active infection, you may also use these preparations for symptom relief. Many of these herbs are available in Oriental food markets, fresh food markets, and health food stores.

The herb yellow dock may be used as an alternative to salt water in nasal irrigation (see pages 89–91). Boil water, then make a mild infusion of yellow dock tea. When the infusion is lukewarm, use it as you would salt water to clear each nostril. Some herbalists recommend alternating between salt water and yellow dock to irrigate a clogged nose.

Echinacea is often recommended by herbalists as an immunity-enhancing herb. It is available in tincture form (drops) or as a loose herb to make into tea. Goldenseal, another powerful herb believed to affect the immune system, can also be taken as a tincture or a tea. When taking herbs in tincture form, pay careful attention to dosing directions and any contraindications on the package.

A variety of other herbs and herbal preparations are available to treat sinus symptoms. If you are seriously considering making herbal remedies part of your daily routine to lessen the severity of sinusitis, it makes good sense to go to the library to read about herbs and to seek the advice of a reputable and experienced herbalist.

Acupressure

Acupressure is a form of Chinese medicine that uses points along *meridians*—invisible lines of energy running beneath the skin—to relieve symptoms of many ills, including sinusitis. Acupressure uses the same points as acupuncture, except that finger pressure, rather than needles, is used to stimulate the points. Here is a brief overview of the acupressure technique that can be used to relieve sinus symptoms:

To start, gently massage around the orbits of the eyes and around the sinus areas. Then locate the pressure points on the face, using the tips of your index fingers. Apply steady pressure for at least three minutes, until you feel the points throbbing. Gently release your fingers from the points.

Pressure points to help sinus symptoms are located

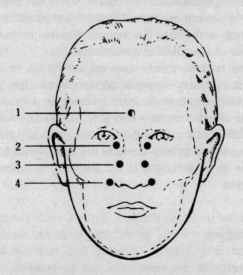

Pressure Points to Relieve Sinus Symptoms

midway between the eyebrows (*1*); in the nasal corners of the eye socket on either side of the bridge of the nose (*2*); along the edge of the nasal bone in the groove along the nose (*3*); on either side of the nose at its widest point (*4*). Another point that helps relieve sinus symptoms (as well as headache, toothache, and other "head" problems) is located in the webbing between the thumb and the index finger.

Relaxation Techniques

As discussed in Chapter 2, for many people stress plays a role in triggering sinus attacks or in worsening the symptoms of chronic sinusitis. Of course, stress can also contribute to general feelings of malaise and interfere with well-being; so reducing the amount of stress in your life makes sense from several standpoints.

Simple relaxation techniques are among the easiest— and least expensive!—ways to decrease stress. Just about any technique can work, from listening to a relaxation tape (the sound of waves breaking on the beach, sounds of a waterfall or rain pattering on trees) to yoga and meditation, to a simple prayer. If you're not accustomed to taking time to relax, try one of the following techniques to get started.

Ten-Second De-Stress Break.   Here's a quick exercise to do during any stressful period: Stop what you are doing. Take five deep breaths, inhaling and exhaling deeply and slowly. At the same time, say to yourself, "R-e-l-a-x," very slowly. Take another deep breath, inhaling and exhaling. Then go back to whatever you were doing prior to taking your de-stress break. Repeat this exercise as often as necessary. If you do it at least ten times daily during stressful periods, this de-stress response can become almost automatic within a few weeks.

Visualization.   Visualization is the process of using your imagination—or "mind's eye"—to form a specific picture of yourself. Chronic sinusitis sufferers can use this technique to imagine the sinuses clear and healthy. While visualization alone won't cure your sinusitis, it can help reduce stress-related sinus attacks. It can also serve as a reminder to take the necessary steps in "real life"—taking medication, using nonmedical techniques—to keep your sinuses as clear as possible.

Start by sitting in a quiet, comfortable spot or lie in bed. Breathe slowly and deeply, becoming as relaxed as possible. Close your eyes and put your imagination to work: Create a picture of yourself feeling healthy, energetic, symptom free. Imagine yourself breathing freely and easily, without a congested nose or clogged sinuses, without headache or sinus pain. See yourself breathing freely in a variety of situations: on the job; at home; during an exercise class; while reading, shopping, watching television. Imagine fresh, clean air filling your nose, lungs, and sinus passages. Put the energy of belief and expectation behind your images, to give them strength and power. Then slowly open your eyes, continuing to breathe slowly and deeply.

This exercise can take as little as five or ten minutes daily. It's a technique that has been shown to be effective in helping many people realize goals (such as weight loss or quitting smoking) and lessen symptoms of disease. Of course, visualization is not a substitute for medical treatment; it is a strategy to try in addition to following an appropriate course of treatment for sinusitis and any related disorder.

Affirmations.   Like visualization, using affirmations—positive thoughts and statements—can act as a form of "self-hypnosis" to put you in a positive frame of mind, reduce stress, and help motivate you to follow the appropriate steps to stay as healthy and symptom free as possible.

The best times to use affirmations are in the morning when you awake and before going to sleep. You can also use them immediately after a negative thought (e.g., "I'm going to have sinus headaches forever") to counteract the self-defeating effects of negative thinking.

Here are several affirmations that may work for you. Use them as guidelines to make your own personal list. Remember that affirmations should be in the present tense, not the future ("I am doing something"—not "I will do something"), so that you feel empowered in the here and now.

• I am eliminating stress in my life every day.

• I am breathing more freely than ever before.

• My sinuses are healing now.

• I allow my mind and body to relax and feel at peace.

• Sinus symptoms are an insignificant part of my life.

IMPORTANT POINTS ABOUT
NONMEDICAL TREATMENT

- Nonmedical techniques are useful in relieving sinus symptoms but not in curing an active sinus infection. These strategies should be used in addition to, not instead of, medical treatment.

- Controlling your exposure to allergens and environmental irritants can help reduce sinus attacks that are associated with allergies and in people who are sensitive to certain irritants in the air.

- Keeping sinuses clear with steam inhalation, saline nasal sprays, and pungent foods can help you breathe easier.

- Following a healthful diet; staying active; and using herbal preparations, acupressure, and stress reduction techniques can help lessen sinus symptoms and improve your health overall.

SHOULD YOU HAVE SURGERY?

Most cases of sinusitis can be treated with medication and by avoiding the precipitating factors discussed in Chapter 2. However, surgery should be considered in three types of circumstances. One, which happens infrequently, is when an acute sinus infection becomes so severe so quickly that complications such as a brain abscess or meningitis threaten to occur (see Chapter 1). In this case, emergency sinus surgery may need to be performed.

Another situation in which surgery should be considered is when your sinusitis does not respond to medication; either it doesn't clear up at all, or it keeps recurring despite your having followed an appropriate course of treatment for sinusitis and for any condition such as an allergy that may contribute to your sinus attacks.

Finally, you may want to consider surgery when sinusitis is clearly due to an anatomic problem such as polyps or a deviated septum, and your symptoms don't clear up with medication.

It's important to recognize that while surgery often improves sinusitis and relieves symptoms, it is not considered a cure. In some cases, full-blown sinusitis may recur even after surgery; in other cases, even though there is significant improvement in sinusitis symptoms, you may still need to take medication to treat acute sinus attacks and continue to use the preventive strategies—medical and nonmedical—described in Chapters 4 and 5.

Several techniques can be used in sinus surgery. The one that is used by a majority of sinus surgeons today, especially for first-time operations, is called *endoscopic surgery.* This technique, which has become increasingly popular in the past decade, generally has fewer complications than more traditional sinus surgery. Because it is the most frequently used procedure, we will cover this procedure in detail.

Since there may be reasons to perform a more traditional type of sinus surgery in selected cases, you should discuss your options during an initial consultation with a sinus specialist. Three of the more traditional approaches —*Caldwell–Luc, external frontal ethmoidectomy,* and *osteoplastic obliteration*—are briefly described later in this chapter (see pages 107–8).

The medical information for the following sections has been provided by David Kennedy, M.D., a pioneer in the use of endoscopic sinus surgery in the United States, and chairman of the department of otorhinolaryngology, head and neck surgery, at the University of Pennsylvania School of Medicine.

Now let's take a closer look at what to expect—and the steps you should take—when undergoing sinus surgery.

SELECTING A SINUS SURGEON

When considering sinus surgery, it's important to select a physician who is experienced in the procedure needed to treat your sinusitis. Endoscopic surgery, for example, requires special training in proper use of the endoscope. Some surgery on the ethmoid sinuses may be performed by using a headlight and microscope inserted through the nose—a technique that is similar to endoscopic surgery but does not offer as much detail in the visualization of the diseased portions of the sinus. This is a technically difficult procedure that also requires a highly skilled surgeon.

In most cases, the sinus surgeon you select will be an *otolaryngologist* (or *otorhinolaryngologist*)—a specialist in ear, nose, and throat disorders. All the qualities described in Chapter 3 for selecting a physician apply to selecting a sinus surgeon. In addition, you should select a surgeon who frequently performs sinus surgery but who also has enough time to oversee your postoperative care. The ideal would be a surgeon who performs an average of five surgeries per week. This person would have enough time in his or her schedule to monitor your recuperation.

Other helpful criteria for selecting a sinus surgeon include making sure the person is board certified by the American Academy of Otolaryngology—Head and Neck Surgery and, if possible, affiliated with a teaching hospital.

THE INITIAL EVALUATION

Once you've decided on a surgeon, it's time to make an appointment for a complete evaluation. For the initial consultation, bring a letter from your physician describing your past history of sinus problems and treatment up until the present time. You should also have a copy of your complete medical history, previous X rays, and results of any other diagnostic tests (described in Chapter 3) that may have been performed.

You will probably be asked to have a CT scan prior to your initial consultation. The results of this test should also be available to help the surgeon make an informed decision regarding the need for surgery.

If, after the consultation, you both agree that surgery may be helpful, an appointment is arranged. Although endoscopic and other types of sinus surgery can be performed on an outpatient basis, many specialists prefer to do the procedure in the hospital so you can stay overnight for observation in case any complications develop (if you have asthma, you should be admitted to the hospital). Follow-up visits are required (described on pages 111–2).

WHAT IS FUNCTIONAL ENDOSCOPIC SURGERY?

As we saw in Chapter 3, an endoscope is a rigid tube that acts like a tiny telescope to give a physician a very detailed view of the area where the sinuses drain into the nose and throat. It can be used for diagnosing the possible cause of sinusitis (e.g., a structural problem in the nose) and for pinpointing the affected sinuses. It is also used to perform sinus surgery.

In functional endoscopic surgery, tiny surgical instruments are attached to the endoscope. It transmits pictures to the physician that enable him or her to maneuver the tiny tools to cut away inflamed or infected tissue. The procedure is called *functional* endoscopic surgery because its purpose is to restore the sinuses' ability to function as close to normally as possible.

Functional endoscopic surgery is a relatively new procedure; it's been in use in the United States only since 1984, although it has been used successfully for a longer period of time in Europe. It differs from traditional sinus surgery in several ways. First, it emphasizes a careful diagnostic workup to identify the affected sinuses. Frequently, the problem is in the area of the ethmoid sinuses —one of the most difficult areas for a physician to see, since they are located deep in the skull, behind the frontal and sphenoid sinuses. In fact, the endoscope permits a physician to obtain the most detailed views of the ethmoids and the other sinuses, both before and during surgery.

Endoscopic surgery can also be less invasive than other types of sinus surgery. In traditional forms of sinus surgery, doctors may make an incision through the upper gum under the lip or near the eye to reach the sinuses, or an incision is made behind the hairline, so the skin can be peeled down to reveal the sinuses. In endoscopic surgery, a tube is inserted through the nose to reach the sinus area.

A main focus of endoscopic surgery is the area near the ethmoid sinuses called the ostiomeatal complex—the place where the sinuses drain into the nose and throat and the part of the sinuses that is most exposed to pollution and allergens and often becomes blocked. If the ostiomeatal complex can be opened up and drainage restored, then more extensive surgery on the sinuses may be avoided.

Because the endoscope can pinpoint inflamed or infected tissue and distinguish it from healthy tissue, the physician can remove only the affected tissue and leave the healthy tissue intact. Endoscopic surgery is also used to remove polyps and correct structural defects in the nose such as a deviated septum and bone spurs.

OTHER SURGICAL TECHNIQUES

If the sinus surgeon you select is not trained in endoscopic surgery, if you have multiple problems that may require very extensive surgery, or if you have had endoscopic surgery and your sinusitis has recurred, you may be a candidate for a more traditional procedure.

Caldwell–Luc

This procedure offers an external approach to the maxillary sinus and is usually performed when an unusual problem, such as a tumor, is causing sinusitis. An incision is made through the upper gum, under the lip, so the surgeon can gain access to the sinus.

External Frontal Ethmoidectomy

In this procedure, the surgeon explores the frontal sinus directly by making an incision from the medial angle of the eye (the point on the nose that is in line with the center of the eye) down along the side of the nose. This procedure is primarily used to improve drainage in the frontal sinus.

Osteoplastic Obliteration

In this procedure, the surgeon opens the front wall of the frontal sinus by making an incision behind the hairline and bringing the skin down over the face. Then the surgeon cleans out the lining of the sinuses, cuts around the bone, and puts fat from the stomach into the sinuses to prevent the cleared areas from refilling with air. This procedure is effective for long-term management of difficult cases of sinusitis that don't respond to other types of medical treatment.

STEPS TO TAKE BEFORE SURGERY

If you smoke cigarettes, you should stop for at least three weeks prior to surgery. As we saw in Chapter 2, smoking cigarettes interferes with the proper functioning of the sinuses. Cigarette smoke introduces toxins into the respiratory tract and also slows down the action of the cilia, the tiny hairlike projections in the lining of the sinuses that sweep mucus out through the sinus ostia.

Not surprisingly, smoking also interferes with the success of sinus surgery. Smoking during the weeks before (or after) sinus surgery can result in excessive scarring and failure of the operation.

Aspirin and any salicylate-containing analgesics should be avoided for at least ten days prior to surgery. Aspirin is an anticoagulant (it keeps blood from clotting); so having aspirin in your system may result in significantly increased bleeding during surgery and in the postoperative period.

Ibuprofen-containing medicines also increase bleeding, but their effect on the blood wears off in a shorter period of time than the effect of aspirin. Medicines with ibuprofen should not be taken for at least five days prior to surgery.

Acetaminophen has no effect on bleeding during or after surgery and may be taken up to the day of surgery.

People who are taking oral steroid medication for asthma or sinusitis should talk with their physician about decreasing the dosage prior to surgery.

In some cases, your sinus surgeon may recommend taking oral steroids or antibiotics prior to surgery to protect against infection.

PRESURGERY TESTS

During the week prior to surgery, you will have blood chemistry tests to determine your overall health status. If you are taking theophylline for asthma, your blood level of theophylline will also be tested.

An *electrocardiogram* (*EKG*) (measurement of your

heart function) or a chest X ray may also be required. If you haven't already had a CT scan of your sinuses, one will be done prior to surgery.

WHAT TO EXPECT DURING ENDOSCOPIC SINUS SURGERY

Functional endoscopic sinus surgery may be performed under local or general anesthesia, with an anesthesiologist standing by to monitor your sedation. Many surgeons prefer local anesthesia because there is less bleeding and there are fewer risks of anesthesia-related complications. Also, when local anesthesia is used, you can give your surgeon feedback if you experience any discomfort or your vision is affected (see "Possible Complications," pages 112–3). However, if you feel you would prefer general anesthesia, discuss this option with your surgeon.

When endoscopic surgery is done with local anesthesia, your nose will be completely numb. You'll probably feel sleepy and relaxed; if you like, you may listen to music on a headset during surgery.

The length of the operation depends on how much work needs to be done to open up the sinus passageways and remove infected tissue (or polyps). Normally, the procedure will last anywhere from one and a half to two and a half hours.

Sometimes, hearing the crunching of bones during surgery can be disconcerting, even when you don't feel any pain. Since you can talk during surgery, you can tell the surgeon if anything bothers you or feels very uncomfortable.

POSTOPERATIVE CARE

Very precise postoperative care is essential to the success of sinus surgery. It's very important to keep all your postoperative appointments and follow instructions carefully; otherwise, extensive scarring, inflammation, or infection may occur, which can cause the sinuses to become blocked. You will probably need to make weekly appointments with your sinus specialist until healing is nearly complete—approximately four to six weeks.

Many patients wonder whether their nose will be packed after surgery. The answer is probably not. In a majority of cases, packing is not necessary. In cases where your surgeon feels packing would be beneficial, small sponges—not the old-style, tight packing with cotton wads—are used. The sponges stay in place for 24 or 48 hours. If your surgery is performed in the hospital, the sponges will be removed before you leave the hospital. If surgery is performed on an outpatient basis, you will have to return to the surgeon's office a day or so after surgery to have the sponges removed.

Part of postoperative care involves cleaning of the area where surgery was performed and removing any scarred or inflamed tissue. During your postoperative visit, your surgeon will apply a topical anesthesia and do a brief endoscopic procedure to clean out the area. Medication may also be prescribed to reduce inflammation and treat or prevent infection.

You will probably have some bleeding from the nose after surgery and after any postoperative cleanup procedures. Plan to be relatively inactive for a week or so (no bending, straining, lifting) and only moderately active until healing is complete (no rigorous exercise is permitted until after the nose and sinuses are fully healed). Other postoperative instructions will be given to you during the initial consultation and after surgery.

The main goal of postoperative care is to prevent a recurrence of sinusitis symptoms—to rout out infection or inflammation, to keep the sinus ostia open, and to avoid blockage. If you wait until you have symptoms again before seeing your physician, then the beneficial effects of surgery may already be lost.

POSSIBLE COMPLICATIONS

All surgery carries with it the possibility of some risks and complications. Fortunately, the risk of serious complications developing from sinus surgery is very low and has been reported to be less than 1 percent.

There are three potentially serious complications of sinus surgery. One is the rare chance of creating a leak of cerebrospinal fluid (the fluid that surrounds the brain) during surgery on the ethmoid sinus. This leak would create a potential pathway for infection, which could result in meningitis. If the surgeon becomes aware of the leak during surgery, a small patch can be placed on the area to allow it to heal. Very rarely, a leak is persistent and may require a second operation.

The other two potentially serious complications concern the eye, because sinus surgery is performed very close to the eye. There is a very rare risk of developing temporary or prolonged double vision or losing vision altogether as a result of sinus surgery. If the surgery is performed under local anesthesia, the vision problem might be restricted to one eye, because you would notice it and immediately tell the surgeon. But if surgery is performed under general anesthesia, there is an extremely rare—less than 1 in a 1,000—risk of losing vision in both eyes. A new device called an *orbital monitor* may help reduce the risk of vision problems during endoscopic surgery by alerting the surgeon to pressure changes in the eye.

The Caldwell–Luc procedure may also cause numbness of the lip, prolonged loss of sensation in the teeth, and rarely, eventual loss of teeth. Traditional procedures may cause more discomfort and swelling than endoscopic surgery, and some minimal scarring.

Other possible risks of sinus surgery are those associated with any type of surgery: adverse reactions to anesthesia (traditional sinus surgery is performed under general anesthesia), risk of infection from a blood transfusion (rarely required for sinus surgery), and risk of infection from viruses or bacteria in the environment.

SURGERY TO REPAIR A DEVIATED SEPTUM

In addition to opening the ostiomeatal complex and removing diseased tissue, it may be necessary to repair the nasal septum during endoscopic surgery. During this procedure, there is a small risk of infection or creating a hole in the septum, which could cause difficulty in breathing through the nose. It's also possible for the cartilage in the septum to shift back during the postoperative period to its original, deviated position, setting the stage for sinusitis symptoms once again.

IMPORTANT POINTS ABOUT
SINUS SURGERY

- Sinus surgery, like any surgery, should be considered a medical treatment of last resort; it is an option for people with chronic sinusitis whose symptoms don't respond to the medical treatments described in Chapter 4. Fortunately, in the vast majority of sinusitis cases, surgery is not required.

- Functional endoscopic surgery is rapidly becoming the surgical procedure of choice for sinus surgery in the United States.

- You should take the same care in selecting a sinus specialist—usually an otolaryngologist or otorhinolaryngologist—to perform sinus surgery that you take in selecting your primary care physician.

- Become aware of all possible risks and complications, as well as potential benefits, of sinus surgery when making your decision.

- If you decide to undergo sinus surgery, be prepared to follow all pre- and postoperative instructions carefully.

SEVEN

CHILDREN AND SINUSITIS

With few exceptions, the causes and symptoms of sinusitis in children are similar to those in adults. However, there may be important differences in diagnosis and treatment, depending on the philosophy of the physician who is managing your child's sinusitis. Some physicians are conservative in their approach, preferring to do as little diagnostic testing as possible and prescribing only those medications they believe are necessary to treat infection; others are more aggressive, ordering tests to help confirm a diagnosis and prescribing medicine for symptom relief as well as to combat infection.

While relatively few scientific studies have been conducted on adults with sinusitis, even fewer have been conducted on children suffering from sinusitis. Most experts agree that further study of the causes, mechanisms, diagnosis, and treatment of sinusitis in children could be helpful in defining strategies that might prevent an acute, first-time sinus attack from developing into recurring, chronic sinusitis.

Such studies could also result in standard guidelines for pediatricians and family practitioners to use in diagnosing and treating sinusitis in children. As it stands now, each clinician is on his or her own in this regard. Some physicians simply extrapolate to children pertinent findings from the limited studies conducted with adults. But others are cautious about translating to children the diagnostic techniques and treatment strategies used with adults—particularly since even studies of adults with sinusitis have not reached clear-cut conclusions. For this reason, selecting the right pediatrician is very important (see pages 119–20 for advice).

DOES YOUR CHILD HAVE SINUSITIS?

Some sinusitis symptoms in children are similar to those in adults—congestion, nasal discharge, bad breath, fever. Headache and facial pain are rare, however, especially in children under age six, in whom the frontal sinuses have not yet fully developed.

As with adults, sinusitis in children most often develops as a consequence of an upper respiratory tract infection such as a cold or flu. Clues that an upper respiratory tract infection may have caused a secondary sinus infection generally occur in two situations: when symptoms persist longer than ten days without improving; or when the upper respiratory tract infection is unusually severe, producing high fever and a thick nasal discharge.

As a parent, you will probably be the first person to recognize sinus symptoms in your child. But this does not mean you should attempt to diagnose or treat the condition on your own. If you are wrong, or if you merely treat symptoms when an underlying infection exists, you may unnecessarily expose your child to the risk of complications from sinusitis (infection spreading to the eyes or brain) or other diseases by delaying appropriate treatment.

If your child's respiratory symptoms persist, worsen, or seem very severe, contact a physician immediately.

CAUSES OF SINUSITIS IN CHILDREN

Many of the causes of sinusitis in children are similar to those in adults. As noted above, the most frequent cause in children is an upper respiratory tract infection that develops into a secondary sinus infection. Children who are allergic or who suffer from asthma are also prone to developing sinusitis.

Environmental irritants such as chlorinated water and dry air produced by certain air-conditioning and heating systems may trigger sinusitis in children. But the most potent environmental pollutant responsible for sinusitis and other respiratory ills in children is *passive cigarette smoke*. Recent studies show that children of parents who smoke cigarettes are many times more likely to develop respiratory diseases and disorders than children of non-smoking parents.

Small children are apt to place a "foreign body" into the nose—that is, an object that fits but doesn't belong there. A foreign object can clog the nose and, by extension, the sinuses.

Congenital abnormalities such as *cleft palate* (incomplete closing of the palate), *choanal atresia* (incomplete opening of the nasal-sinus passage), *pharyngeal stenosis* (narrowing of the pharynx), and *adenoid hypertrophy* (overgrown adenoids) can interfere with proper respiration and predispose children to sinusitis. As with adults, a deviated septum, a tumor, or dental problems can also lead to sinusitis in children.

Relatively rare congenital systemic disorders such as *cystic fibrosis* (a metabolic disorder) and *immotile cilia syndrome* (a condition in which the sweeping movement of the cilia is impaired) may predispose children to sinusitis. And as with adults, children who have diseases that weaken the immune system are more likely to experience sinus disorders than children who are healthy.

Sinusitis and Asthma

Sinusitis in children may trigger asthma attacks, just as it does in adults. Therefore, any child with a history of asthma also should be examined for sinusitis. If sinusitis is diagnosed, it should be treated promptly.

A recent study published by the American Lung Association revealed that childhood asthma has increased by more than 30 percent in the past decade, from 2.4 million children in 1980 to 3.7 million in 1992. Possible reasons for the increase include many of the factors that also cause sinusitis: indoor air with high concentrations of irritants and allergens, pollutants in the environment, and cigarette smoke. The researchers speculate that rapid spread of upper respiratory tract infections in day care settings may also make some susceptible children more prone to developing asthma or asthmalike symptoms.

DIAGNOSING SINUSITIS IN CHILDREN

As noted above, physicians may differ in their approach to diagnosing and treating sinusitis (and other childhood disorders, as well). Many will attempt to diagnose sinusitis in children on the basis of symptoms, a physical examination, and medical history rather than subjecting children to X rays or other diagnostic tests at the outset. They will order such tests only if symptoms persist or worsen after appropriate treatment.

Other physicians may order diagnostic tests immediately or may refer a child to a specialist. As noted above, there is no universally accepted protocol, or management strategy, for sinusitis. Because of these differences, you may want to spend time interviewing and selecting a doctor for your child as you would for yourself.

Selecting the Right Doctor for Your Child

The criteria outlined in Chapter 3 for selecting a physician also apply to selecting a pediatrician or general practitioner to treat your child. Ask for recommendations, talk with the physician's staff, and set an "interview appointment" to meet with the physician directly.

When others recommend a pediatrician to you, the American Academy of Pediatrics (see "For More Information," page 136) suggests you ask the following questions:

____ Are all of your questions answered by the pediatrician and the office staff?

_____ Do you think your children respond well to the doctor?

_____ Does the pediatrician seem to know the latest advances in pediatric medicine?

_____ How helpful and friendly are the office staff?

_____ How well does the office staff manage your phone calls?

_____ If an emergency arises, how is it handled?

_____ Do you regularly experience long delays before seeing the pediatrician?

_____ Is there anything about the pediatrician (or the office) that troubles you?

During your meeting with a prospective pediatrician, ask whether he or she is certified through the American Board of Pediatrics and also a member of the American Academy of Pediatrics. These professional societies require members to meet professional standards.

If your child has a history of sinus and respiratory problems, ask whether the physician is knowledgeable about diagnosing and treating sinusitis in children. Try to determine whether the doctor's approach is conservative or aggressive (see page 119) and decide which management style you would prefer for your child.

Of course, the bottom line is that you—*and* your child—feel comfortable with and trust the physician.

The Initial Diagnosis

As noted earlier, many physicians prefer to make an initial diagnosis of sinusitis based on a review of your child's symptoms, medical history, and a physical examination. If after treatment sinus symptoms persist or worsen, additional diagnostic tests may be ordered.

Symptom Review

Congestion, nasal discharge, bad breath, and fever are the hallmark sinus symptoms in children. Some or all may be present. As with adults, these symptoms are nonspecific, meaning they are also common to other diseases and disorders such as a cold or flu. But if such symptoms persist for more than ten days or are very severe at the outset of an upper respiratory infection, then sinusitis may be suspected.

Medical History and Physical Examination

During the medical history, your child's physician should be informed of any prior history of sinus disease and how it was treated. If you or other members of your family seem prone to sinusitis or other respiratory problems, this fact should be noted as well. While there are as yet no scientific studies showing that a propensity toward sinusitis may be inherited, many physicians believe that sinus disorders, like asthma and allergies, tend to "run in families."

Your child should then have a physical examination, including listening to the heart and lungs, examining the eyes and ears, examining the nose and throat, and examining the lymph nodes in the neck and under the arms for evidence of a systemic infection. In children over age ten, transillumination—shining a light across the maxillary and frontal sinuses to see how much light is reflected through onto the palate—may also be useful in confirming a diagnosis (see Chapter 3 for more details).

If after reviewing symptoms, taking a medical history, and performing a physical examination the physician believes your child has sinusitis, he or she may begin treatment immediately or order additional tests to confirm the diagnosis.

Additional Diagnostic Tests

The role of X rays in diagnosing sinusitis in children is controversial. Some physicians do them routinely; others hesitate to expose children to X rays unless absolutely necessary and may order them only if medical treatment fails to resolve sinusitis, or if a structural abnormality is suspected. This is an issue that should be discussed with your child's physician, preferably *before* a sinus problem arises.

As we saw in Chapter 3, CT scans of the sinuses produce more clearly defined images of the sinuses than X rays. However, some pediatricians believe their use should be reserved for the evaluation of recurrent, chronic sinus infections, rather than using them to evaluate a single, acute sinus attack. Again, this is a matter of professional judgment—but it underscores the importance of giving your child's physician a complete medical history. If a doctor is unaware that your child has had sinus attacks in the past, he or she may assume the attack that brought your child to the office was a one-time event.

Endoscopy is difficult to do with children and takes a high degree of skill. As of this writing, it is not commonly used by pediatricians or general practitioners to diagnose sinusitis in children; your child's physician should refer you to an ear, nose, and throat specialist with training and experience in endoscopy (see "Selecting a Sinus Surgeon," page 104) to perform the procedure in cases where sinusitis is difficult to diagnose or is unresponsive to medical treatment. Other visualization techniques such as MRI and ultrasound are not recommended.

Antral puncture—inserting a needle-type tool into the maxillary sinuses through the nose or through the lip and aspirating out fluid for culture—is reserved for very severe cases of sinusitis that aren't resolved after treatment or for cases in which complications, such as eye infection or brain abscess, are suspected. Your child would be referred to an ear, nose, and throat specialist for this procedure. As with selecting any physician, it's a good idea to talk with the specialist in advance to make sure he or she is experienced in doing antral puncture.

Taking a nasal smear—looking at tissue from the nose under a microscope—is of limited value in children. The microorganisms that are discovered in the nose are not necessarily the ones that are infecting the sinuses. If a physician suspects an unusual organism is infecting the sinuses, an antral puncture will probably be recommended instead.

If an allergy is suspected, your child will be referred to an allergist or immunologist for testing. The procedures used would be the same as for adults: skin or blood testing, food challenge, pet challenge. These tests are described in Chapter 3. If a dental problem is believed to be causing sinus symptoms, your child will be referred to a dentist or endodontist.

A diagnosis of nonallergic rhinitis is difficult to make. You and your child would have to be very aware of the situations in which sinus attacks developed and try to make some connection between the attacks and environmental irritants.

Other rare causes of sinusitis in children such as systemic disease and immune dysfunction would be diagnosed using an array of tests, and in consultation with specialists in the areas in which the disease is suspected.

TREATING SINUSITIS IN CHILDREN

Studies have shown that as many as 40 percent of children recover spontaneously from an acute sinus attack— that is, they recover without taking medication. However, no studies have documented the rate of recurrence of sinusitis in these children or established whether they go on to develop chronic sinusitis. Therefore, most physicians would prefer to treat a sinus attack medically in the hope of completely clearing the sinuses of infection and preventing recurrence.

Nonmedical strategies can be helpful in preventing recurrent, noninfectious sinus attacks and in lessening symptoms when such attacks do occur. Or they can be used in conjunction with medication during an active sinus infection. As with adults, these strategies are especially important when sinusitis is associated with allergies or irritants in the environment.

Medical Treatment

The objectives of medical treatment of sinusitis in children are the same as those for adults: to control infection; to reduce swelling of the mucous membranes in the nose and sinuses, thereby clearing the sinus ostia; and to ensure that the sinuses remain unclogged and infection free for as long as possible. Medical treatment would also include treating any underlying diseases or disorders such as allergy that may be triggering sinusitis.

As with adults, antibiotics are the mainstay of treatment for sinus infection in children (see Chapter 4 for an overview of prescription and nonprescription medications used in treating sinusitis and related disorders). Amoxicillin is the antibiotic of choice because it tends to be effective in a majority of cases, has relatively few side effects in children, and is inexpensive. If your child is sensitive to penicillin, trimethoprim/sulfamethoxazole will probably be prescribed. Any of the other antibiotics used for adults may also be prescribed, depending on the judgment of your child's physician.

There are no universally accepted guidelines for types of medications to be used in sinusitis in children or duration of treatment. Many physicians will prescribe antibiotics for ten days to two weeks and then check to see whether symptoms have been completely resolved. Others will keep treating until all symptoms are resolved, then treat for an additional seven days.

No studies have demonstrated the effectiveness of other medications such as decongestants, corticosteroid sprays, or analgesics in treating sinus symptoms in children. Most physicians agree that antihistamines should not be used unless your child has a proven allergy. The other medications may be prescribed at your physician's discretion, depending on the severity of your child's symptoms. Many physicians would encourage the use of nonmedical techniques such as nasal irrigation or saline nasal sprays instead of drugs to treat symptoms.

Medical treatment for conditions that predispose to sinusitis, such as allergies, environmental irritants, nasal obstructions, and systemic disorders, would be similar to the treatment prescribed for adults, described in Chapter 4.

Sinus Surgery

In children, sinus surgery is usually the medical treatment of last resort. Because there is a good chance that children will "outgrow" many or all of their sinus symptoms—that is, symptoms may lessen or disappear altogether as the immune system develops—most physicians will advise treating symptoms medically and waiting to see what happens before suggesting surgery.

If sinus surgery is performed on a child, it will be done under general anesthesia. The techniques would be similar to those described in Chapter 6. After surgery, a second visit to the surgeon's office would probably be needed to clean out any remnants of diseased tissue. Contrary to the treatment of adults, the cleaning process in children would also be done under general anesthesia to eliminate discomfort and ensure that the child remains still during the procedure. Additional follow-up visits would be scheduled to monitor the healing process and make sure that no infection develops.

Nonmedical Techniques

The nonmedical strategies used to control sinusitis symptoms in children are mostly the same as those you would use to control your own sinusitis symptoms, described in detail in Chapter 5. However, there are some additional points to bear in mind. By now, you are probably aware that if your child's sinusitis appears to be linked to allergies or asthma, *environmental control* is very important. But it's important to remember that your child may spend a good deal of time in several different environments, not just the home environment.

The school your child is attending should also be examined for allergy, asthma, and sinusitis triggers. You should meet with school personnel—teachers, nurses, administrators—to devise strategies to minimize your child's exposure to these allergens. Your child's physical education teacher should also be alerted to the possible impact of exercise on your child's sinus condition, especially if the indoor environment is lacking in ventilation. School personnel should also be made aware of any medications your child is taking that might affect school performance or behavior.

Other "environments" include facilities used for after-school activities, as well as homes of friends and relatives. Similar discussions should be held with people in these places, as well.

Nonmedical strategies to clear the sinuses are particularly important for children when decongestants are to be avoided. You may wish to purchase a humidifier to keep sinuses moist. Although you can adapt the nasal irrigation techniques described in Chapter 5 for use by children, it's easier to purchase or prepare a saline nasal spray that can be conveniently used to help clear congestion.

Staying healthy by following a healthful, balanced diet and exercising regularly is as important for your child as it is for you. Whether herbal preparations or acupressure techniques should be tried is up to you (if you purchase herbs in tincture form, read labels carefully for contraindications in children).

As noted in Chapter 2, the role of stress in triggering sinus attacks is controversial. However, some pediatricians believe that parents may be too quick to dismiss a child's symptoms as "all in your head"—particularly nonspecific symptoms such as fatigue and head or facial pain. It's important to note that even if sinus symptoms are triggered by stress, they are not any less "real" than if they are triggered by a viral infection. As one pediatrician put it, "Every child has a weak spot"—a part of the body that is more prone to respond to stress than others. If sinuses are your child's "weak spot," the symptoms they cause should still be treated, if not with medicine, then with nonmedical strategies.

If your child appears receptive to doing relaxation exercises such as those described in Chapter 5, by all means encourage their practice. Beyond possibly relieving sinus symptoms, such strategies can help your child maintain a more peaceful state of mind—a benefit to everyone!

IMPORTANT POINTS ABOUT CHILDREN AND SINUSITIS

- The causes and symptoms of sinusitis in children are similar to those in adults. But differences may arise in diagnosis and treatment, depending on the philosophy of your child's physician.

- In children, the most common sinusitis symptoms are congestion, nasal discharge, bad breath, and fever. Head and facial pain are rare.

- The most common cause of sinusitis in children is an upper respiratory tract infection that doesn't get resolved. Other causes include allergies, sensitivity to irritants in the environment, placing a foreign object in the nose, and congenital disorders. Children with asthma should also be examined for sinusitis, since sinusitis can trigger asthma attacks.

- Diagnosis and treatment of sinusitis in children may differ among doctors. Some physicians aggressively use diagnostic tests and medicines; others are more conservative. Most pediatricians attempt to diagnose sinusitis based on your child's symptoms, medical history, and physical examination. Sinus X rays or other tests might be ordered to confirm a diagnosis.

- Any condition predisposing to sinusitis such as allergy

or structural or systemic problems must also be treated.

- Nonmedical techniques such as controlling environmental allergens and irritants, using saline nasal sprays, eating right, and exercising regularly can be very effective in controlling sinus symptoms with or without medication.

EIGHT

LIVING WITH SINUSITIS

By now, you've probably realized that chronic sinusitis, like most chronic disorders, waxes and wanes at different times. Sometimes its symptoms become severe and may require prompt medical attention; at other times, you may scarcely be aware of any symptoms at all. What accounts for such variations?

A large part of the answer depends on *you*. Certainly, some people are more prone to sinusitis and respiratory problems than others, though scientists don't yet know why. Being one of those people with a sinus "weak spot" is something you simply need to accept.

But that doesn't mean you have no control over your sinusitis; to the contrary. You've learned in this book that the vast majority of sinus attacks that cause debilitating congestion, nasal discharge, fatigue, head and facial pain, and an overall clogged-up feeling are triggered by an upper respiratory infection, allergy, or irritants in the environment. In many instances, these are triggers you *can* do something about!

The first thing you can do is stay as healthy as possible. Eating right, exercising regularly, and reducing stress in your life—in other words, taking care of your physical and emotional health—can help keep your immune system strong. This can reduce your chances of developing the illnesses that may predispose you to sinusitis.

If your sinus attacks occur in association with allergic reactions, you can take steps to eliminate these allergens from your life as much as possible. The same goes for irritants, especially cigarette smoke. Steer clear of the substances that irritate your nose and sinuses, and you will go a long way toward lessening the impact of sinusitis in your life. As we'll see below, creating a plan of action to systematically reduce these triggers can give you a good deal of control over your sinusitis.

Do you have to take sinus medication every day for the rest of your life? In most cases, the answer is no. Of course, you've learned that if your sinuses become actively infected, the infection should be treated with medicine to decrease the chances of severe complications. But on a daily basis, there are a whole range of nonmedical techniques described in this book that can help you keep sinus symptoms to a minimum much of the time.

The bottom line is that you can live with sinusitis, and live well and comfortably, without resorting to drastic measures to reduce your symptoms. You can play a major role in helping to prevent sinus attacks, and in seeing to it that the attacks that do occur are relatively mild, by incorporating some changes into your life-style.

CREATE AN ACTION PLAN

Start taking charge of sinusitis by creating a plan of action to stay healthy and reduce as many of the sinus attack triggers in your life as possible. This process is really useful for everyone: We can all benefit from following a healthful life-style and keeping our environment as clean and irritant free as possible.

1. *Review your diet.* Are you eating a variety of foods? Are you getting all the nutrients recommended for good health? If certain foods such as dairy products cause congestion, have you identified satisfactory alternatives? Consider working with a registered dietitian or other health professional with nutrition expertise to develop a healthful eating plan.

2. *Take a careful look at your environment,* which includes your home, office, your child's school, and any other place in which you or your children spend a significant amount of time. Start by keeping your home clean, and allergen and irritant free, using the techniques described in this book.

   Next, evaluate other environments. Initiate a meeting at work to discuss ways of keeping the office free of allergens and irritants. Have similar discussions with personnel at your child's school.

   Be aware of the air quality at your gym or health club. If necessary, talk with personnel in these places about the need for proper ventilation and the importance of reducing dust in the air and of keeping floors, carpets, equipment, and pool water clean.

3. *Review your life-style habits.* If you smoke cigarettes, quit now. Cigarettes harm your health overall and impair the cilia in your sinuses. Passive smoke inhaled by your children can predispose them to sinus attacks.

Be aware of how alcohol affects your sinus symptoms. You may experience congestion as a result of additives in certain types of alcoholic beverages (e.g, sulfites in wine).

4. *Incorporate regular exercise into your life.* You'll feel better, look better, and probably breathe better, too (people with asthma should create an exercise program with a physician's guidance).

5. *Learn to relax.* Many people believe that stress can act as a trigger for sinus attacks and other ills. *Relax*—and you're likely to feel better and function better in all aspects of your life.

MAINTAIN A POSITIVE ATTITUDE

Probably the most important thing you can do to lessen the effects of sinus symptoms is to believe the above strategies really can make a difference. Don't give in to defeatist thinking or feel like a victim of sinusitis. Current thinking about chronic illness is that your attitude *does* matter. While positive thinking alone can't cure sinus disease, it can motivate you to take all the steps in your power to lessen the severity of symptoms and the frequency of sinus attacks.

If your sinusitis is associated with allergy and asthma,

consider joining a support group where you can share your experiences and knowledge with others. For more information about a group in your area, contact the Asthma and Allergy Foundation of America, listed in the next section.

IMPORTANT POINTS ABOUT LIVING WITH SINUSITIS

- You don't have to be a victim of sinus disease. You can take control of many of the factors that trigger sinus symptoms, minimizing their impact.

- Staying healthy, eliminating allergens and irritants from your environment, and reducing stress in your life can go a long way toward decreasing the frequency and severity of sinus attacks. In many instances, you will need medication only during active sinus attacks and to treat any disorder that triggers sinusitis.

- Maintaining a positive attitude—truly believing in the power of the steps you are taking to keep sinusitis under control—will keep you motivated over the long term.

By using the information in this book, selecting a knowledgeable physician to treat and monitor sinus attacks, and enlisting whatever other support you need, you can join the millions of sinusitis sufferers who have learned to control their symptoms and enjoy life more than ever before.

FOR MORE INFORMATION

American Academy of Allergy and Immunology (AAAI)
611 East Wells Street
Milwaukee, WI 53202
(414) 272-6071

AAAI offers a toll-free physicians' referral and information line: 1-800-822-ASMA. The organization also publishes a newsletter and literature on sinusitis and allergies.

American Academy of Otolaryngology—Head and
  Neck Surgery
One Prince Street
Alexandria, VA 22314
(703) 836-4444

This organization offers free brochures on sinusitis, postnasal drip, hay fever, and other related disorders.

American Academy of Pediatrics (AAP)
141 Northwest Point Boulevard
Post Office Box 927
Elk Grove Village, IL 60009-0927

Write to the AAP for brochures and information on selecting a pediatrician and parenting advice. You may also take advantage of the AAP's pediatrician referral service by sending a stamped, self-addressed envelope and a letter indicating the cities in which you would like pediatricians identified.

Asthma and Allergy Foundation of America (AAFA)
1125 Fifteenth Street NW, Suite 502
Washington, DC 20005
(202) 466-7643

AAFA has a toll-free number for information about asthma and allergic disorders: 1-800-7-ASTHMA. The organization also publishes a monthly newsletter and informative brochures.

National Institute of Allergy and Infectious Diseases
National Institutes of Health
9000 Rockville Pike
Rockville, MD 20892
(301) 496-4461

This federal agency is responsible for much of the research related to allergic diseases and can provide information on sinusitis as well.

National Jewish Center for Immunology and
   Respiratory Medicine
1400 Jackson Street
Denver, CO 80206
(303) 388-4461

The National Jewish Center has a toll-free information line called LUNG LINE, staffed by registered nurses who answer questions, send literature, and give callers advice about allergies, lung diseases, and immunologic disorders. Call 1-800-222-LUNG.

GLOSSARY

allergen   Any substance capable of causing an allergic reaction in susceptible people. Examples include dust mites, molds, and animal danders.

allergic reaction   An immune response that takes place following repeated contact with an allergen.

analgesic   Medication used to treat pain. An analgesic may be used if sinusitis symptoms include head or facial pain.

antibiotic   Medication used to treat infection. Antibiotics are the mainstay of treatment for sinus infection.

antihistamine   Medication that blocks the effects of histamine, a chemical released in response to an allergen. Antihistamines are used to treat symptoms of allergic rhinitis, such as sneezing and itchy, watery eyes and nose.

antral puncture   A diagnostic technique used when sinusitis fails to respond to conventional medical treatment or when an unusual organism is suspected of causing infection. A physician inserts a needle-type tool into the maxillary sinuses through the nose or through the lip.

asthma A disease characterized by narrowing of the bronchial tubes and accompanied by wheezing or shortness of breath. More than half of asthma sufferers also have sinusitis. Sinusitis is believed to trigger asthma attacks.

choanal atresia A congenital disorder that results in incomplete opening of the nasal-sinus passage.

cilia Hairlike projections in the lining of the sinuses that sweep mucus out into the nose and throat. When the sinuses become infected and inflamed, the sweeping movement of the cilia decreases or may even stop altogether.

computed tomography (CT) scan The diagnostic test of choice for confirming a diagnosis of sinusitis. It produces clear pictures of the sinuses using a much lower dose of radiation than conventional X rays.

corticosteroids Synthetic hormones that are used in antiinflammatory medicines. Corticosteroid nasal sprays are used to reduce swelling and inflammation of the mucous membranes of the nose.

dander Bits of cells and debris from animals and insects that may cause an allergic reaction when inhaled by susceptible individuals.

decongestant Medication used to shrink swollen nasal membranes, promoting the free flow of air through the nose and sinuses. It is available as a topical nasal spray or drops, or in tablet, liquid, or capsule form.

endoscopy The use of a tube that acts like a tiny telescope to help diagnose sinusitis or to perform sinus surgery.

food challenge A test used to determine whether a person is sensitive or allergic to a specific food. In a double-blind food challenge, suspect foods and neutral, or placebo, foods are put into opaque capsules or puddings. They are then swallowed by the person being tested. Neither the patient nor the physician knows which capsules or puddings contain the suspect food and which ones contain the placebo. If a person has an allergic reaction to a suspect food under these conditions, a cause-and-effect relationship between the food and the reaction may be established.

histamine A chemical released in response to an allergen. Histamine is considered responsible for much of the swelling and itching symptoms of an allergic reaction.

immune system The cells and chemicals that work to protect the body from potentially infectious microorganisms such as bacteria, viruses, and fungi.

immunotherapy Regularly injecting solutions of symptom-causing allergens into the body in carefully monitored quantities until allergic reactions no longer take place.

irritant Any substance that irritates the nose, eyes, or sinuses and causes symptoms. An irritant is different from an allergen in that it does not trigger an immune response in the body.

magnetic resonance imaging (MRI) A diagnostic technique that provides cross-sectional images of different parts of the body without using X rays or other radiation. MRI is not used for diagnosing sinusitis, except in rare cases when an individual has a severe systemic disease such as cancer or a fungal sinus infection is suspected.

mucoevacuant   Medication that helps rid the body of excess mucus. Also known as an *expectorant*.

mucous membrane   The soft skinlike layer that lines many of the body's cavities and tubes, including the nose, sinuses, and other parts of the respiratory tract. The mucous membrane secretes mucus, the liquid that helps keep these structures moist and well lubricated.

nasal irrigation   A technique that uses salt water to clear the nasal and sinus passageways.

ostiomeatal complex   The space where the sinuses drain into the nose and throat. It is the area that is most easily clogged by nasal and sinus reactions to allergens and irritants. Sinus surgery focuses on opening up this area to restore drainage.

otolaryngologist   A specialist in disorders of the ear, nose, and throat. Also known as an *otorhinolaryngologist*.

polyp   A balloonlike swelling in the nose that impedes free breathing, causing stuffiness and congestion.

radioallergosorbent test (RAST)   A type of blood test used in allergy testing.

rhinitis   Inflammation of the lining of the nose. May be caused by allergies (*allergic rhinitis*), infection (*infectious rhinitis*), or irritants (*nonallergic rhinitis*).

rhinovirus   The family of viruses responsible for causing the common cold.

sinus   A sinus is a hollow air space, of which there are many in the body. The paranasal sinuses—the ones affected in sinusitis—are named for the bone or bones in which they lie. The frontal sinuses are located in the brow area, directly over the eyes. The maxillary sinuses are inside each cheekbone. The ethmoid sinuses are located right behind the bridge of the nose, and the sphenoid sinuses are just behind the ethmoids, in the upper part of the nose.

sinusitis   Inflammation of the sinuses triggered by infection, irritants, allergens, structural problems, dental problems, or systemic disease.

steam inhalation   A technique used to reduce congestion in the nose and promote the free flow of air through the nose and sinuses.

transillumination   A diagnostic test for sinusitis, useful in detecting gross blockage of the sinuses. A physician shines a light across the maxillary or frontal sinuses and sees how much light is transmitted through the palate and back into the mouth.

upper respiratory infection   An infection, usually caused by bacteria or viruses, of the throat, larynx, nose, or sinuses.

INDEX

Marilynn Larkin is an award-winning medical journalist whose articles have appeared in a wide range of national consumer magazines and medical trade publications. She is a contributing editor for *Nutrition Forum,* a former contributing editor for *Health* magazine, and author of *What You Can Do About Anemia* (Dell Medical Library). Marilynn Larkin lives and works in New York City.

QUANTITY SALES

Most Dell books are available at special quantity discounts when purchased in bulk by corporations, organizations, or groups. Special imprints, messages, and excerpts can be produced to meet your needs. For more information, write to: Dell Publishing, 1540 Broadway, New York, NY 10036. Attention: Special Markets.

INDIVIDUAL SALES

Are there any Dell books you want but cannot find in your local stores? If so, you can order them directly from us. You can get any Dell book currently in print. For a complete up-to-date listing of our books and information on how to order, write to: Dell Readers Service, Box DR, 1540 Broadway, New York, NY 10036.